Bike Paths

OF CONNECTICUT & RHODE ISLAND

A Guide to Rail-Trails & Other Car-Free Places

STUART JOHNSTONE

Conditions and information change over time so comments and corrections are appreciated. Address them to:

Active Publications
P.O. Box 1037
Concord, MA 01742

Published by: Active Publications
P.O. Box 1037, Concord, MA 01742-1037
www.activepublications.net

Printed in the United States of America

Publisher's Cataloging in Publication Data

Johnstone, Stuart A.
Bike Paths of Connecticut & Rhode Island: A Guide to Rail-Trails & Other Car-Free Places / by Stuart A. Johnstone; photographs by the author.
ISBN 978-0-9627990-2-0
1. Bicycle touring - Connecticut - Rhode Island - Guidebooks 2. Connecticut - Description and travel 3. Rhode Island - Description and travel
Library of Congress Catalog Card Number: 2012904220

Dedicated

to the many forms of human-powered travel,
and to the people and places that inspire it.

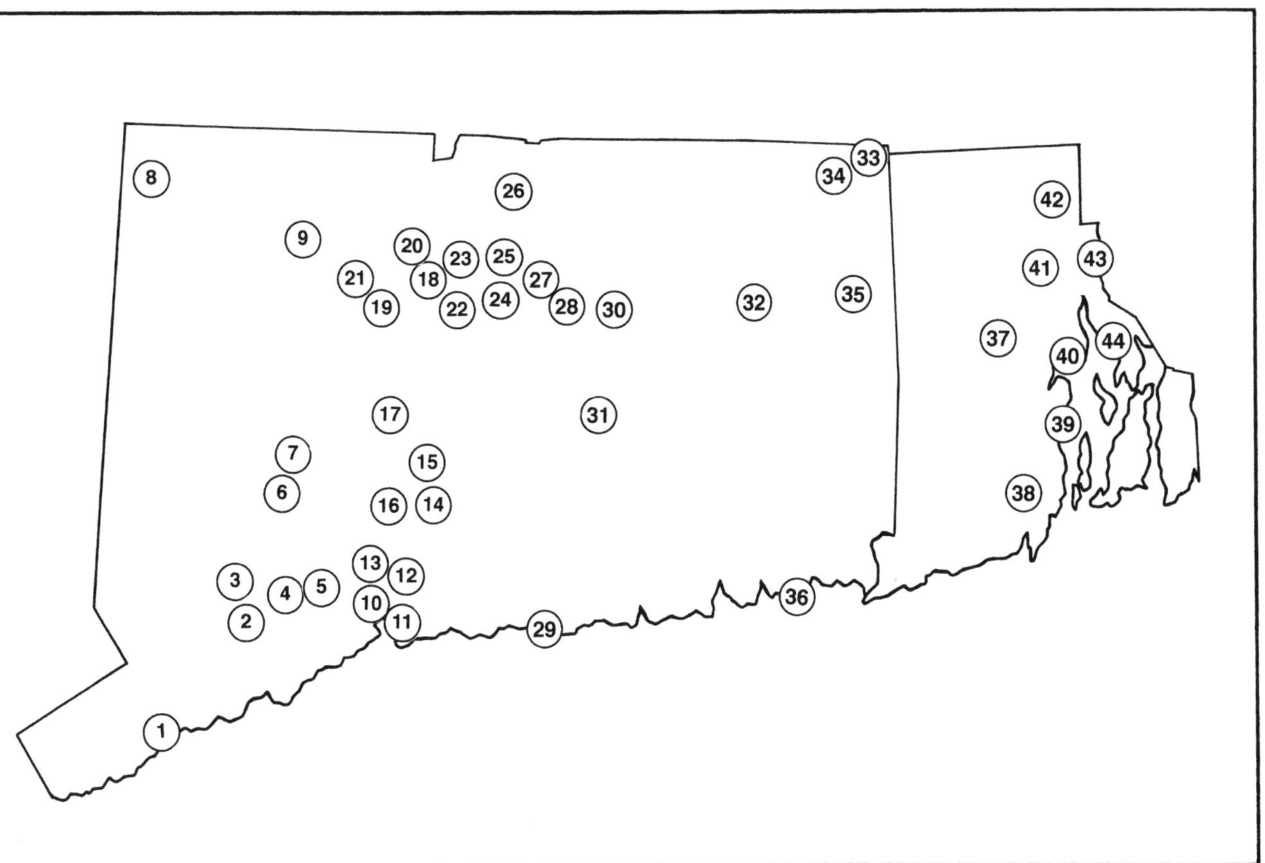
8
26
34
33
42
9
20
23
25
43
21
18
27
41
19
22
24
28
30
32
35
37
44
40
17
31
39
7
15
6
38
16
14
13
12
3
4
5
36
10
2
11
29
1

Contents

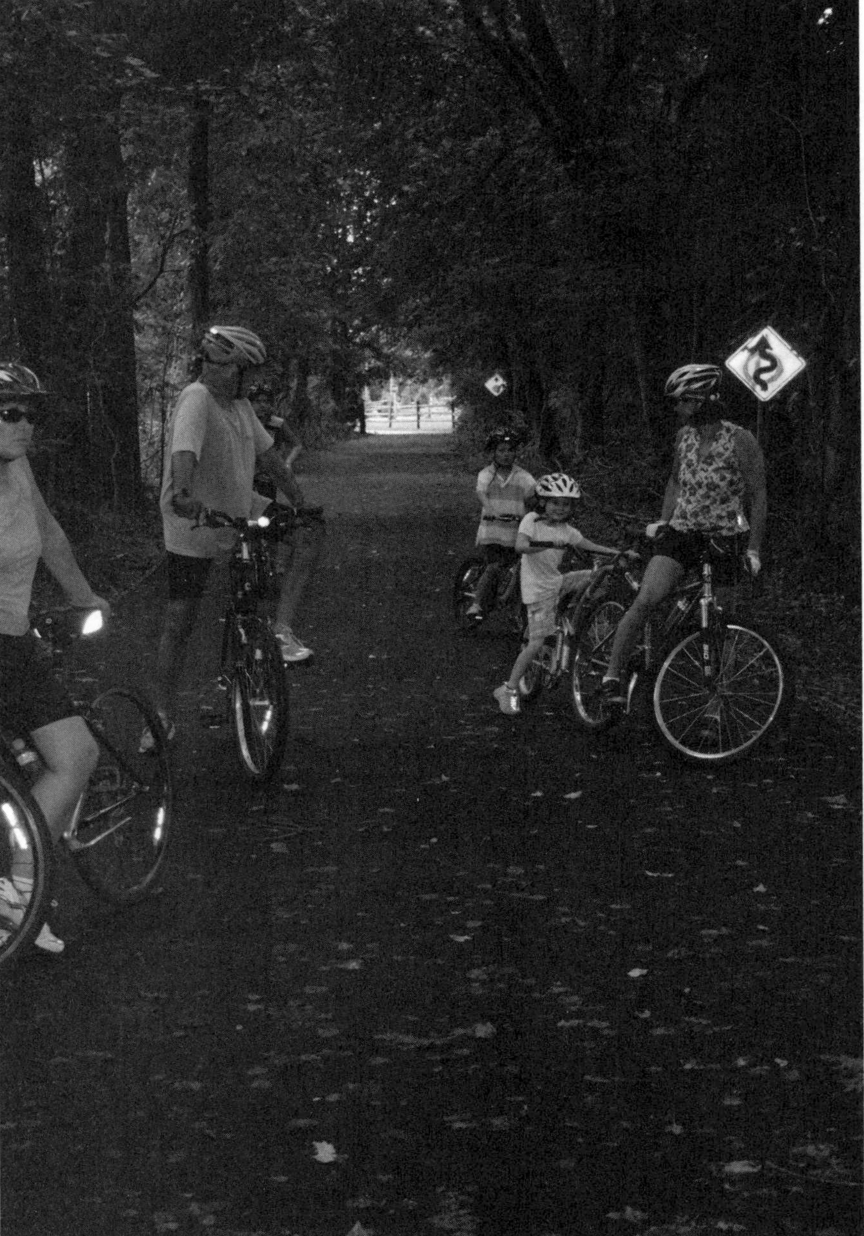

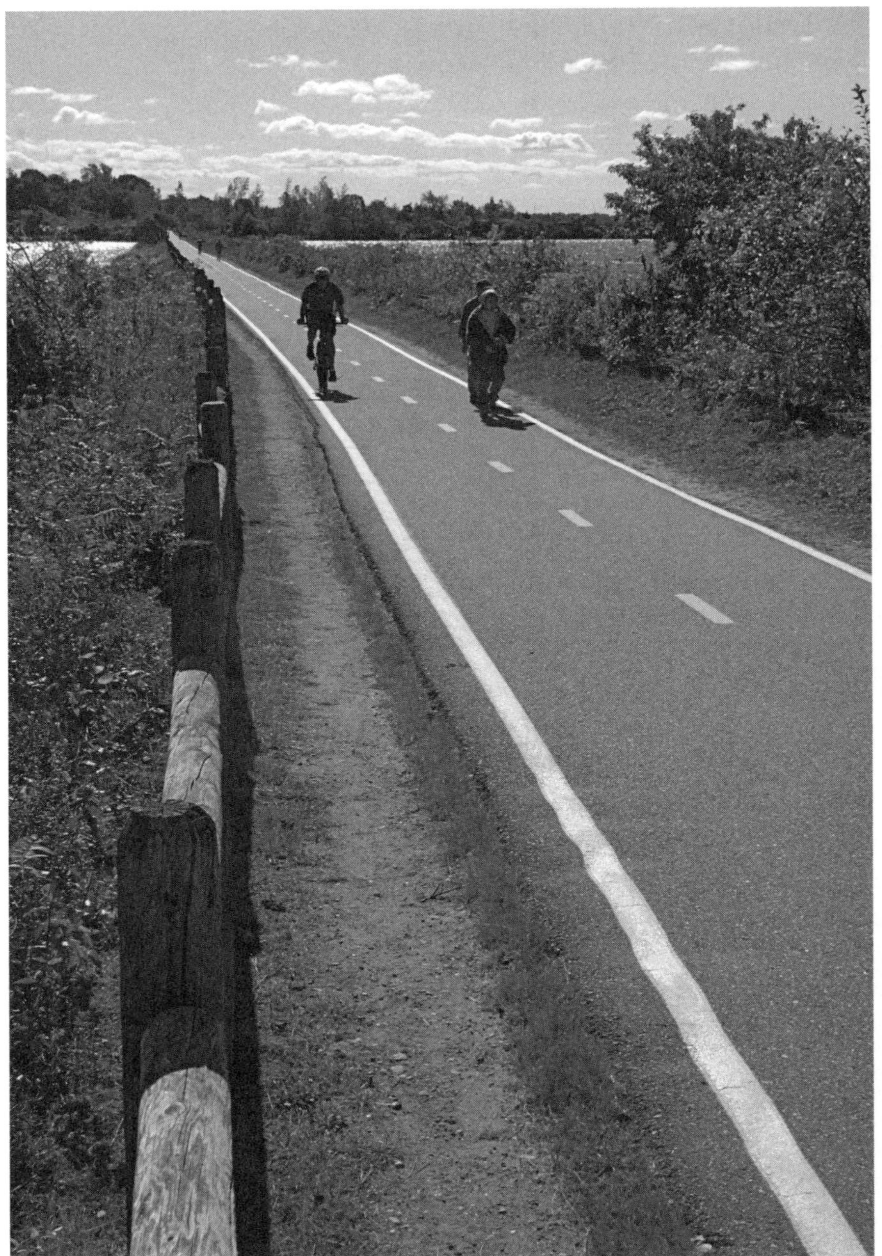

Introduction

Bike paths are special places. Separated from car traffic, their smooth surfaces deliver much more than the people which they carry. Bike paths enhance communities, and regions, with safe bicycle and pedestrian travel, enjoyable places to recreate, motivation to exercise, access to nature, and car-free connections between places. Travel a trail and you are apt to feel free from your stresses, appreciate and enjoy your activity, and say hello to strangers as they pass. And bike paths are places for everyone: all ages and abilities can participate.

New England's diverse and growing network of bike paths, both paved and unpaved, is an increasingly popular resource for recreation and transportation. Connecticut and Rhode Island have created an impressive collection ranging from convenient locations in or near urban areas to completely rural settings. Many are flat, easy routes along former railroads which have been transformed into "rail-trails" creating linear parklands and linking surprisingly distant places. Others follow canal towpaths, former carriage roads, or free-flowing courses through a variety of landscapes in state parks and other public lands. The most popular paths attract steady streams of human-powered traffic but others venture through remote woodlands with plenty of solitude.

Bike Paths of Connecticut & Rhode Island has been written from the bicyclist's perspective but in-line skaters, walkers, and cross country skiers will also find the information useful. A primary objective of the book is to communicate rules and regulations, standards of etiquette, and safety features for the trails since each location has its own set of conditions. It is hoped that readers will appreciate the diversity of options in Connecticut and Rhode Island and be able to plan their rides accordingly.

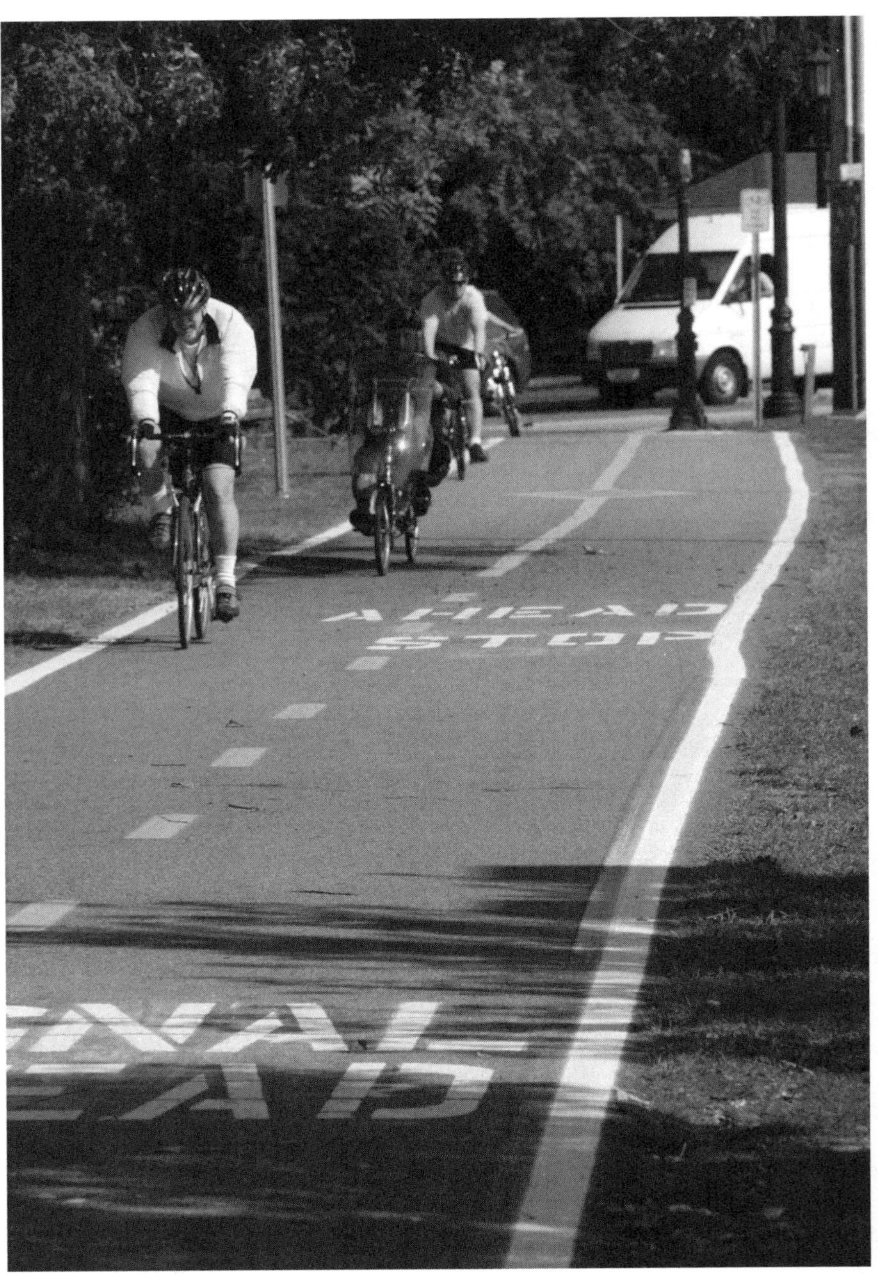

Rules of the Bike Path

1. **Keep to the right.** Most bike paths have two-way traffic so stay on the right side to allow safe passage. Remember that others might need to pass you.
2. **Pass on the left after signaling audibly.** Make verbal contact (*"On your left..."*) or signal with a bell to avoid startling the slower traveler. Look both ahead and behind before passing.
3. **Yield to pedestrians and horseback riders.** Bicyclists and in-line skaters are expected to yield to slower travelers.
4. **Stop at road crossings and look both ways.** Drivers will not always be aware of bike path crossings so assume that they do not see you.
5. **Stay alert and be predictable.** Anticipate the actions of others and let them anticipate yours by avoiding sudden changes in movement. Use extra caution when children and pets are present.
6. **Do not block the bike path when stopped.** Step off the surface to allow others to pass unimpeded.

Both Connecticut and Rhode Island require that ages 15 and under wear approved helmets. All ages should be reminded that serious injuries are possible on bike paths and that the risk of accidents increases in the presence of children, pets, groups of people, multiple activities, and intersections. Bicyclists, because they travel relatively quickly and quietly, present an extra risk for collisions.

Bike paths are not meant for speed. Cyclists planning on riding fast should either use roads or take care in choosing an appropriate place and time.

Noise and litter have a negative impact for other bike path users and for abutting property owners. Respect the

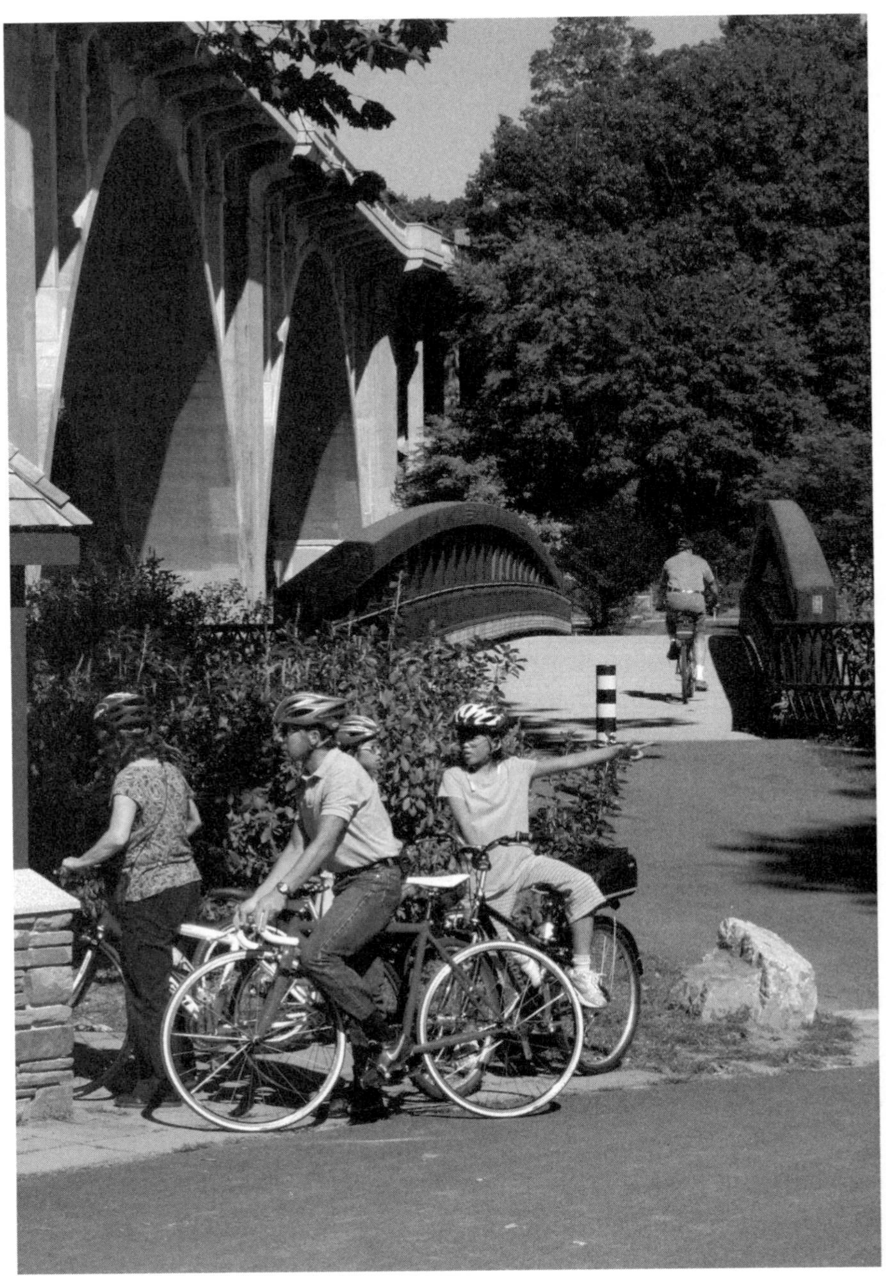

environment of the trail so that others can also enjoy it.

Hunting occurs near bike paths in some areas. The most active hunting period is deer season in the late fall, when trail users are encouraged to wear an article of "blaze orange" clothing. Hunting is not permitted on Sundays in both Connecticut and Rhode Island.

Pet owners should be aware of local leash laws and rules regarding animal wastes. Owners are required to remove their pets' wastes at most trails.

When parking, avoid leaving valuables in your car, even if it is locked. Park at designated locations and be careful not to block trailhead gates because work crews and emergency vehicles always need access.

Planning Your Trip

Be prepared! Getting lost or injured, underestimating trip length or difficulty, and overestimating your own strength or skill level can bring undesireable consequences. A weather change or equipment failure can ruin an otherwise wonderful time. Be ready for unwanted surprises by planning ahead and bringing some useful items.

Drinking water is one of the most essential things to remember, especially in summer. It is easy to become dehydrated while exercising so carry a water bottle or two on the bike or on your body and start drinking before you get thirsty. Longer tours require greater amounts.

Even if you are not planning a picnic, bring something to eat on longer excursions in case your body runs low on energy. A snack can give an important boost both physically and psychologically.

If you are unsure of the trails that you plan to explore, carry a map and keep track of the features that you pass such as road intersections, bridges, and bodies of water. A bicyclist can track mileage using a cyclometer which mounts on the handlebars and displays distance, time, speed, and other information.

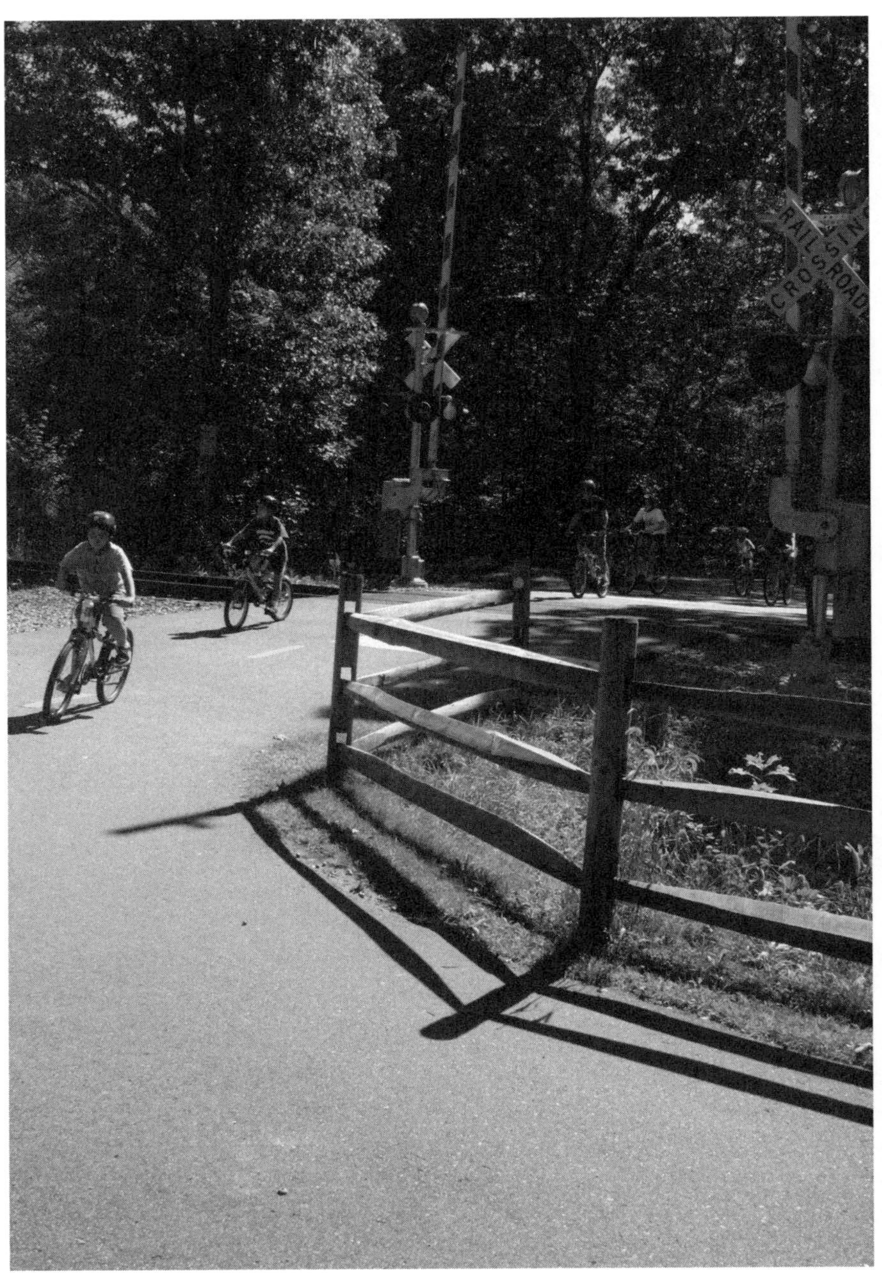
RAILROAD

Bicyclists should consider bringing tools for simple repairs. Since many of the bike paths described in this book reach isolated places, riders will have an important advantage in being able to fix a flat tire or repair a simple mechanical problem. Common supplies include either a spare inner tube or patch kit, a pump, tire irons to remove the tire from the rim, an adjustable wrench, a screwdriver, spoke tightener, and chain tool. These can be carried in a small tool pack attached to the bike frame. If you are not capable of making general bike repairs on the trail and are not self-sufficient with tools, it is wise to ride with others who are.

Other useful items include bug repellent during spring and summer when mosquitos, deer flies, and other insects can create unwanted memories, and extra clothing to suit possible weather changes. First aid supplies are also wise. These items add minimal weight relative to their potential reward.

For safety, ride with a companion and leave word of your planned route with a responsible person.

What to Wear

If you are traveling on wheels, the most important item is a bike helmet. Light and comfortable to wear, it should be worn by all ages as valuable protection from the ground, trees, and other objects encountered along a trail. State laws in both Connecticut and Rhode Island require bike helmets for ages 15 and under. Since three quarters of all bicycle-related deaths result from head injuries, wearing a helmet is a healthy habit. In-line skaters are also encouraged to wear knee, elbow, and wrist protection.

Wear comfortable clothing and dress in layers to allow time to warm up and also to suit possible weather changes.

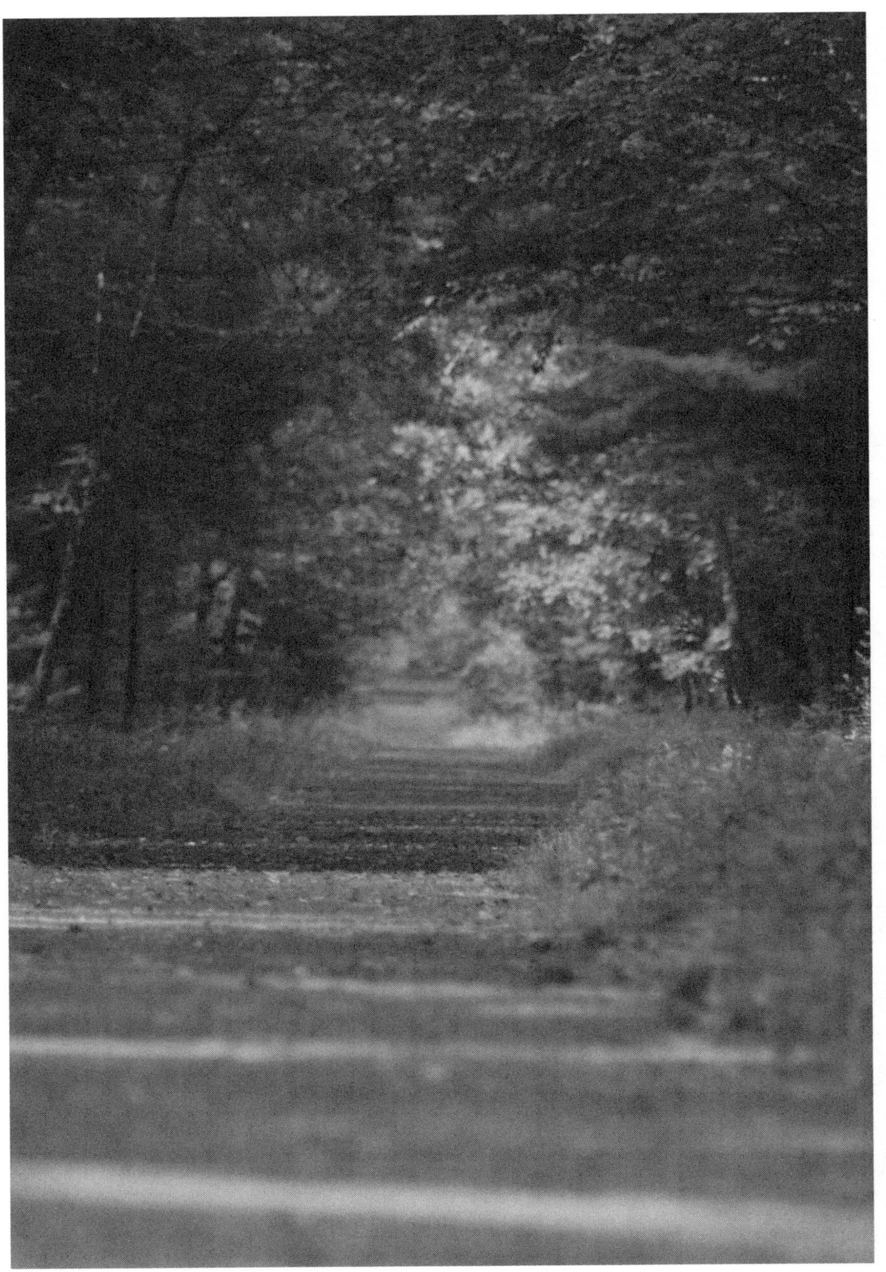

About This Guidebook

Bike Paths of Connecticut & Rhode Island is meant to be a starting point, a means for people to discover a place for themselves. It has been written to prepare readers with rules, trail descriptions, and suggested destinations so that they can better enjoy their explorations. Narrated directions should be recognized as only one of perhaps several ways to tour an area.

Maps are provided to give a general view of trail networks and natural features. Note that the map scale for each area varies widely so plan your distances and courses carefully. The names of trails, roads, and surrounding landmarks appear with boldface type in the text for quick referencing. Only the major parking areas are designated on maps so smaller spots might also exist.

Background information includes pieces of local history for each bike path. Much of the railroad history regarding rail-trails originates from *The Rail Lines of Southern New England* (1995, Branch Line Press, ISBN 0-942147-02-2), by Ronald Karr.

Practical information accompanies each description. This includes the locations of toilet facilities when present and sources of additional information. Driving directions originate from nearby highways and will be most helpful when used together with a road map.

Since improvements to the region's bike paths are on-going, be aware that the length, surface, and other amenities of some trails might be better than they are described in this book.

Get involved!

Plenty of bike path projects could use your help. If possible, volunteer your time and/or money for the benefit of a favorite or a future trail in your area and be a part of the progress.

1 Norwalk River Valley Trail

Norwalk, CT

LENGTH: 1.9 miles
SURFACE: paved
TERRAIN: small hills

Destined to extend northward, this pocket-sized bike path provides enjoyable pedaling through parks near the heart of the city. Highway noise is never far away.

RULES & SAFETY:

- Bicyclists should yield to pedestrians.
- Keep to the right side, ride at a safe speed, and alert others (*"On your left..."*) when approaching from behind.
- Use extra caution when children and pets are present.
- Pets must be leashed and their wastes removed.

ORIENTATION:

The trail's condition and terrain vary: the northern half is new and flat, the southern half is older and hillier. Note that the large, busy intersection of West Ave. lies in between.

TRAIL DESCRIPTION:

Begin at the **Maritime Aquarium** trailhead where trails lead in several directions. Turning right (south), the trail leads for a short distance along the **Norwalk River** to a viewing deck built over the water. Heading straight (east) over a pedestrian bridge, a 0.6-mile loop explores **Oyster Shell Park** where a former landfill has been transformed into hillside greenspace above the river. This loop starts along the water with overgrowing vegetation and corroding asphalt surface, turns and climbs beside **I-95** to the top of the hill for good view, then ends with a short descent.

Here the main trail intersects, linking the aquarium trailhead parking lot (to the left) with points north (to the right). Turning right, cyclists pass under I-95, turn left on **Science Rd.** and cross the railroad, then turn immediately right on **Crescent St.** Just ahead, turn left at the entrance to

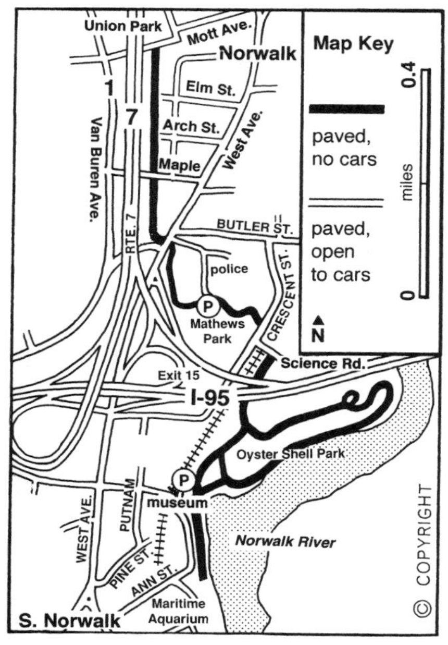

Mathews Park where the trail winds uphill through a playground. Flattening, it continues past parking lots for the police station and childrens museum, skirts the grounds for the **Lockwood-Mathews Mansion Museum**, then reaches the mansion's gatehouse (now visitor information) beside **West Ave.**

Look for the trail continuing diagonally across West Ave., and use appropriate caution when crossing this broad and busy street. The remaining half-mile of trail straightens along a green passageway between the embankment for **Rte. 7** and a residential neighborhood, crossing two more streets before ending at **Union Park** near **Mott Ave.**

BACKGROUND:

The idea of a 20-mile multi-use trail linking Norwalk with Danbury was first proposed in 1970, and construction of Norwalk's first section took place in 2001. The trail threads an intricate course beside the waterfront, a railroad, two highways, and other roads while joining public parks and a former railroad bed. The city plans to eventually extend it northward to the Wilton town line.

DRIVING DIRECTIONS:

From I-95, take Exit 14 if northbound or Exit 15 if southbound. Following signs for the Maritime Aquarium, take West Ave. south to a traffic signal, fork left on N. Main St. and take the next left on Ann St. Continue to the river, curve left, and park in the trailhead lot on the right.

TOILETS:

museums, visitor information center, and police station.

ADDITIONAL INFORMATION:

Norwalk Parks and Recreation: (203) 854-7806

2 Housatonic Rail-Trail

Trumbull, CT

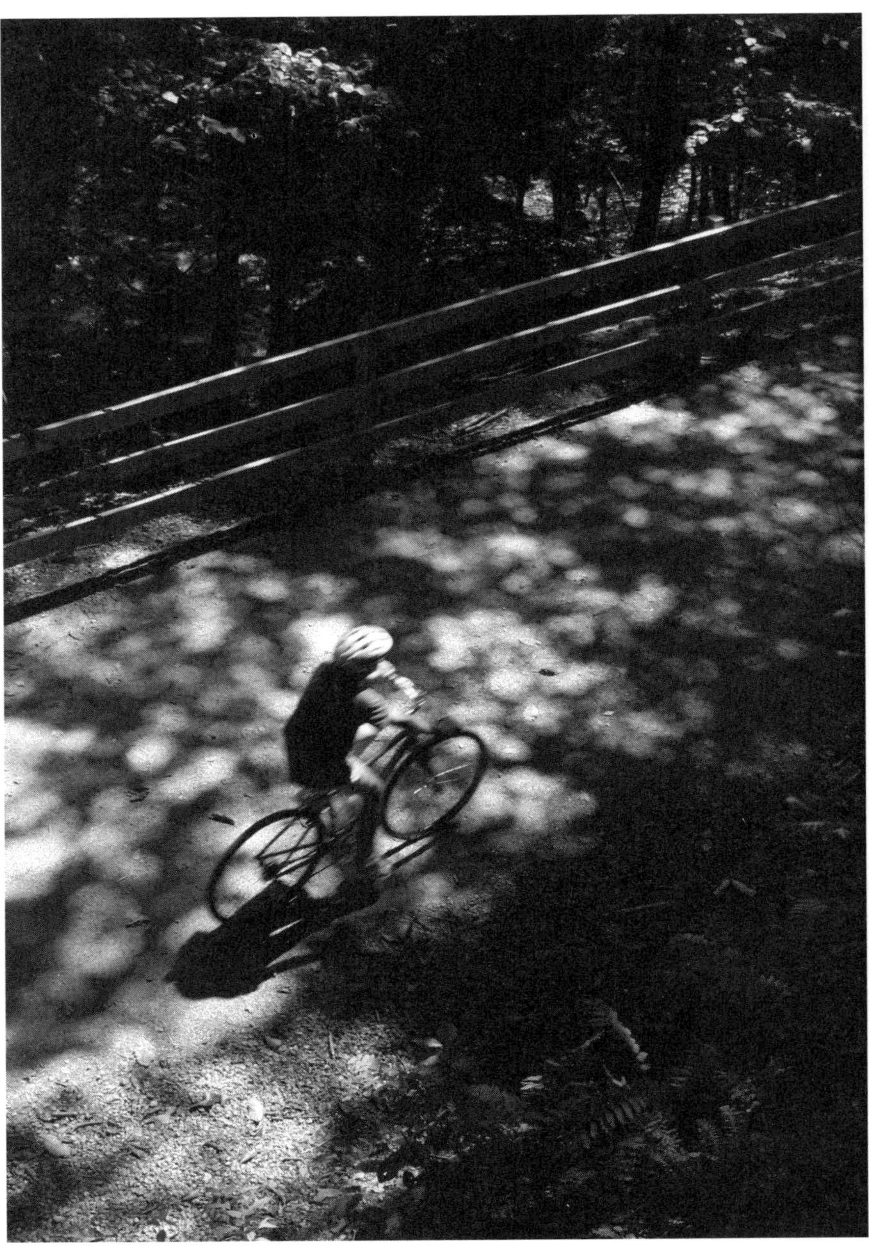

LENGTH: 5.2 miles
SURFACE: half is paved, half is stone dust or smooth dirt
TERRAIN: flat, with small hills at detours from rail bed

Trumbull's surprisingly secluded rail-trail lets bicyclists and others soak up great natural scenery beside the steep, ledgy banks of the Pequonnock River.

RULES & SAFETY:

• Bicyclists should yield to pedestrians and horses.

• When encountering horses, stop at the side of the trail and make verbal contact with the rider so that the animal will feel safe.

• Bicyclists are specifically asked to be courteous. Ride at a safe speed, keep to the right, pass on the left, and alert others (*"On your left..."*) when approaching from behind.

• Hunting is permitted in the area from mid-October through late-December (although it is prohibited by state law on Sundays). If possible, wear blaze orange clothing then.

• Dogs must be leashed and their wastes removed.

• The park closes at sunset.

ORIENTATION:

The trail runs in a mostly north-south direction along a former rail bed following the Pequonnock River. Two detours from the rail bed present hillier conditions, especially near the north end of the trail where a mile-long side trip encounters significant slopes.

The most popular stretch of trail is the southernmost 3.5 miles from Tait Rd. to Old Mine Park. Most of this is unpaved but the surface allows easy riding on stone dust and smooth dirt. Three trailheads serve this distance and the natural scenery ranks among the trail's best.

TRAIL DESCRIPTION:

Starting from **Tait Rd.** at the southern trailhead for the **Pequonnock River Valley Park**, the first half-mile of the rail bed heads north between two residential neighborhoods. It then enters natural surroundings following a shelf of land on a steep slope with the Pequonnock visible and audible below

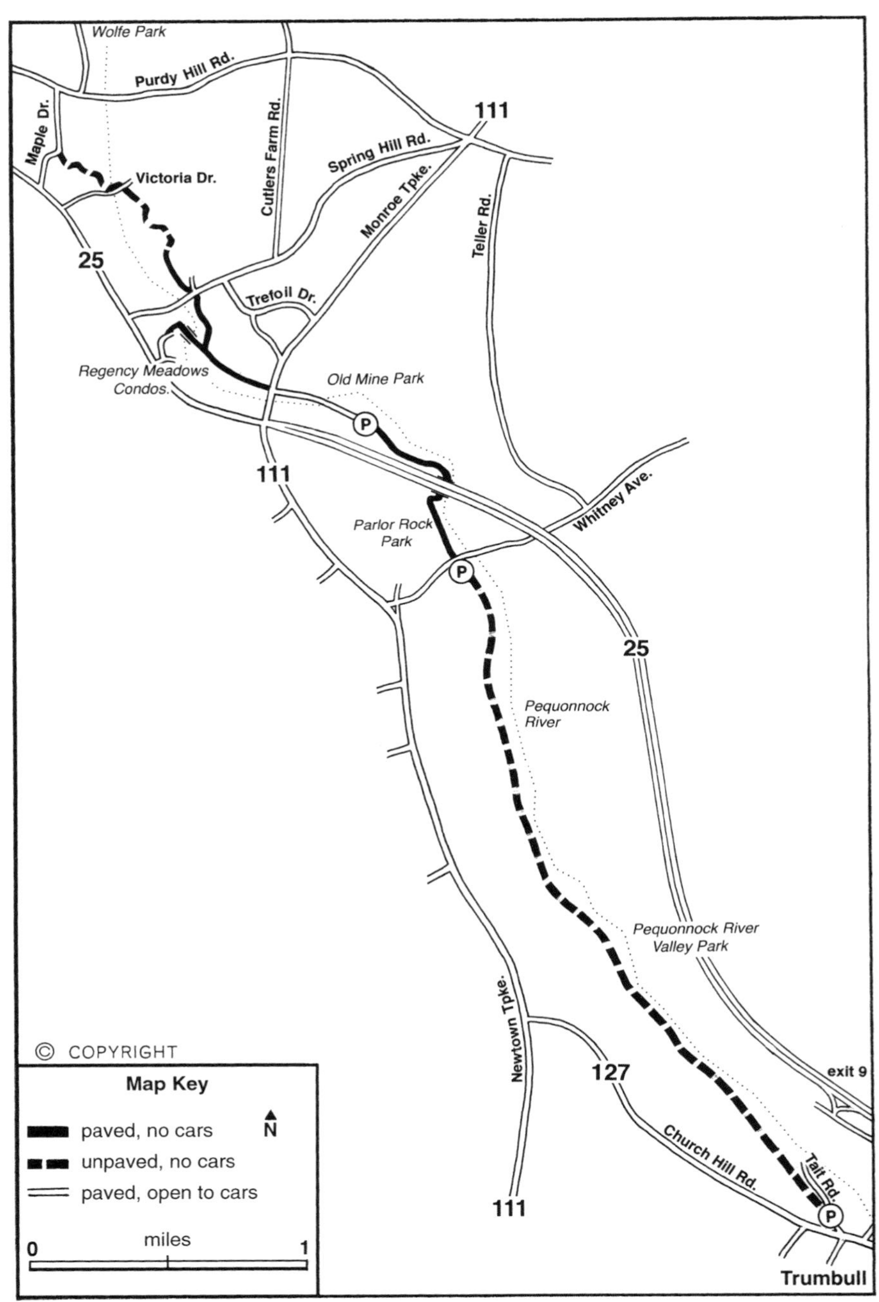
Wolfe Park
Purdy Hill Rd.
Maple Dr.
Cutlers Farm Rd.
111
Spring Hill Rd.
Victoria Dr.
Monroe Tpke.
Teller Rd.
25
Trefoil Dr.
Regency Meadows Condos.
Old Mine Park
P
111
Whitney Ave.
Parlor Rock Park
P
25
Pequonnock River
Pequonnock River Valley Park
Newtown Tpke.
127
exit 9
Church Hill Rd.
Tait Rd.
P
111
Trumbull
© COPYRIGHT
Map Key
paved, no cars
unpaved, no cars
paved, open to cars
N
miles
0
1

the trail on the right side. The river and its rapids are a captivating sight along this stretch especially at several rocky, narrow points along its flow.

The trail continues northward with a faint uphill grade, curving with the contour of the hillside and leaving sight of the river at numerous points. A few wet spots on the surface slow the pedaling but the biking is otherwise easy. Side paths drop to the river and connect the park's other trails for hiking and mountain biking.

About 1.3 miles from Tait Rd., look on the right for the stone foundation of the Old Trumbull Ice House, built to store ice before the days of refrigeration. Ice was harvested in winter beside this building from a reservoir which also provided water for Bridgeport in the 1800's and early 1900's.

After 2.3 miles the trail narrows from overgrowing foliage in a semi-open are, passes a residence on the right side, then emerges at a trailhead parking area on **Whitney Ave.** (2.7 miles). The trail intersects the road at a sloped curve, so use caution when crossing.

Continuing northward, the trail surface has been improved with asphalt for the next several miles. The trail passes **Parlor Rock Park**, site of a late-1800's amusement park which was built by the railroad to attract passengers. A set of prominent ledges and a small gorge in the river make it an interesting spot to rest. Just ahead, **Rte. 25** obstructs the original rail line so the trail makes a 0.3-mile detour by climbing a slope, passing under a highway bridge which spans the river, and then curving through woods on the other side to rejoin the rail bed.

In a short distance, the trail reaches **Old Mine Park** where a trailhead parking lot, small pond, and picnic area await. Owned by the town of Trumbull, this park was the site of an 1800's-era tungsten mine and remnants of the operation are still visible from trails which explore the nearby woods.

Follow the park's entrance driveway to **Rte. 111** (3.9 miles from the Tait Rd. trailhead). After crossing the busy road, the trail enters woods with a paved surface which soon forks. Heading straight, the trail crosses a bridge over the river and follows the original railroad grade for a quarter-mile, then turns left (west) to reach the **Regency Meadows Condominiums**.

Forking right, it begins a mile-long detour from the rail bed by climbing a slope and descending the other side to **Spring Hill Rd.** After crossing this street, look for the trail forking left at an entrance road. The surface reverts to stone dust after a short distance and the trail curves downhill to an office park where it intersects **Victoria Dr.** and crosses the Pequonnock River. It then climbs back to the rail bed, enters woods, and continues with an unimproved surface for a short distance before ending at an elbow turn on **Maple Dr.**, 5.2 miles from the Tait Rd. trailhead.

Exiting onto Maple Dr., turn right (north) to reach the Monroe section of the Housatonic Rail-Trail (Chapter 3). Follow Maple Dr. for two tenths of a mile, turn right on **Purdy Hill Rd.**, and ride downhill for a short distance to the entrance to **Wolfe Park**, on the left. The next section of rail-trail starts ahead on the left side.

BACKGROUND:

The route originated in 1840 as the Berkshire Railroad linking Bridgeport and New Milford, then was purchased by the Housatonic Railroad and eventually became part of the New York, New Haven, and Hartford Railroad. Use of this segment of the rail line declined during the Great Depression and ceased in 1941.

The Bridgeport Hydraulic Company owned and managed much of the surrounding acreage as watershed land from the 1880's until 1989 and prohibited any access to the area. Today the state of Connecticut owns this acreage, known as Pequonnock River Valley Park, and manages it in partnership with the town of Trumbull for recreation and conservation. The Housatonic Rail-Trail serves as the park's main trail, a highlight for many of the park's visitors but merely a starting point for others eager to explore the area's more challenging paths.

Development of the rail-trail has spread northward through other areas of Trumbull in recent years. Future construction could link the Monroe portion of the Housatonic Rail Trail (Chapter 3) in the north as well as Bridgeport in the south.

DRIVING DIRECTIONS:

Tait Rd. trailhead: From Rte. 15 (Merritt Pkwy.), take Exit 49 and follow Rte. 25 north to Exit 9. Follow Daniels Farm Rd. south toward Trumbull for a half-mile to the end, then turn right on Rte. 27 north. After a short distance turn right on Tait Rd. and park ahead at the side of the road, being careful not to block traffic.

Old Mine Park: From Rte. 15 (Meritt Pkwy.), take Exit 49 and follow Rte. 25 north to the end of the divided highway. Turn right on Rte. 111 and look for the park entrance a short distance ahead on the right. Park at the end.

TOILETS:

none provided

ADDITIONAL INFORMATION:

www.gbrpa.org/Regional%20BicycleTrail.html

3 Housatonic Rail-Trail

Monroe, CT

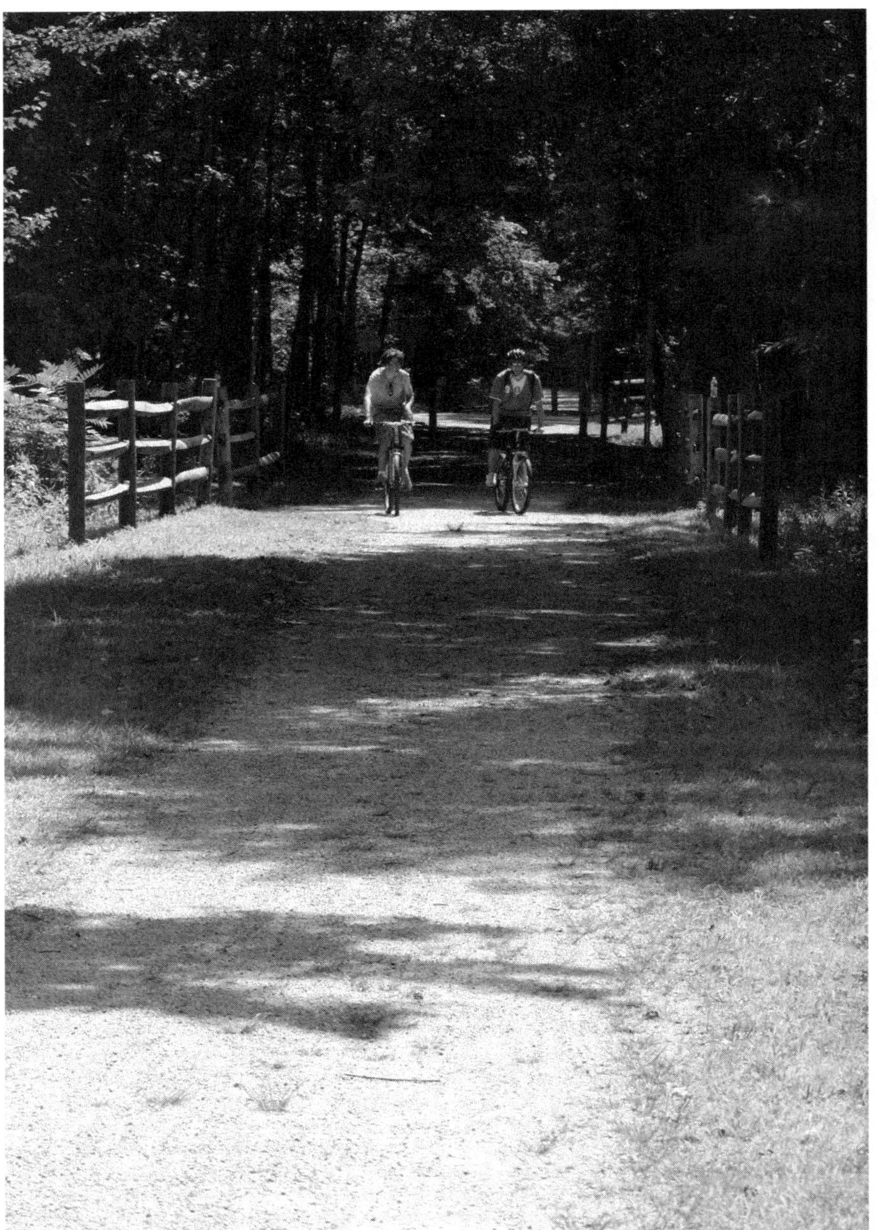

LENGTH: 3.7 miles, (including 0.7-mile detour on roads)
SURFACE: hard-packed gravel
TERRAIN: flat

Monroe's rail-trail quietly slips through town with easy biking on a broad, smooth surface and lots of leafy scenery.

RULES & SAFETY:

• Bicyclists should yield to pedestrians.

• Keep to the right, pass on the left, and alert others (*"On your left..."*) when approaching from behind.

• Be especially cautious in the presence of children and pets since their movements can be unpredictable.

• Step off the trail when stopped so others can pass.

• Use care when crossing roads. Stop before entering the roadway and assume that drivers do not see you.

• Bicycles are prohibited from the trails in the Great Hollow Lake area at Wolfe Park.

• Horses and motorized vehicles are prohibited.

ORIENTATION:

The trail follows a railroad bed for most of the 3.7 mile distance from Wolfe Park in the south to the Monroe/Newtown border in the north with a trailhead parking lot located near the midpoint. A 0.7-mile on-road detour is a minor disruption near the midpoint. The most popular section is the southern portion between the trailhead and Wolfe Park.

The trail is not paved but provides safe, easy biking conditions and a well-groomed appearance. The surface is wide and has borders of mowed grass on each side with wooden fencing for protection where steep bankings or other hazards exist. Road intersections have crosswalks, metal posts to block vehicle entry, and stop signs to warn trail users. Mileage markers beside the trail originate on Purdy Hill Rd. at the entrance to Wolfe Park.

TRAIL DESCRIPTION:

Starting at the **Cutler's Farm Rd.** trailhead parking lot, turn left on the trail and follow it south across Cutler's Farm Rd. The 1.3-mile trip begins with a gentle left-hand

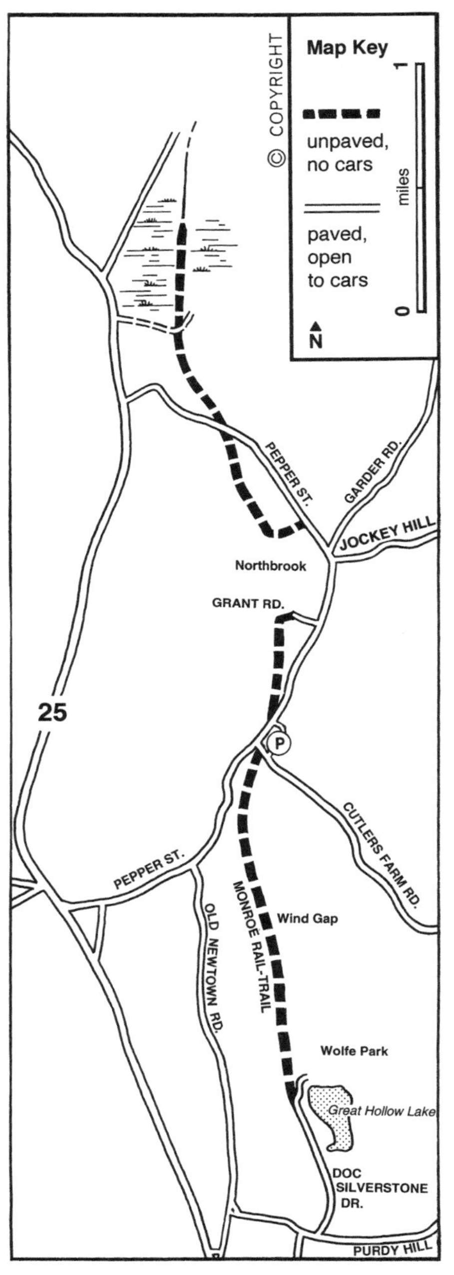

bend on a low, earthen causeway built through a wooded wetland. After three quarters of a mile, riders will notice that the scenery changes dramatically when the trail enters the **Wind Gap**, a 150-foot-deep pass between two hills which is lined with steep slopes, ledges, and boulders.

Slicing through this opening, the trail hugs the right-hand slope as the passage widens into a small stream valley and develops a slight downhill grade which lasts for the remaining half-mile to **Doc. Silverstone Dr.** and the entrance to **Wolfe Park**. Benches are stationed beside the trail at this southern terminus with a view over the swimming beach at **Great Hollow Lake**. Bicyclists should note that the trails exploring Wolfe Park are reserved for foot travel only.

Turning north (right) from the Cutler's Farm Rd. trailhead parking lot, the rail-trail extends for 2.4 miles to the border of Newtown. It crosses **Pepper St.** almost immediately and follows the edge of several fields for a half-mile, then abruptly turns right on a 0.7-mile detour from the rail bed where the **Northbrook** residential development has blocked the original rail bed. Marked by *Bike Route* signs, the detour begins at the end of **Grant Rd.**, turns left on Pepper St. and continues for 0.4 miles, then turns left on a trail that rises on a small hill and returns to the rail bed.

Continuing northward, the rail-trail runs for a half-mile to another intersection with Pepper St., crossing a bridge over a stream and passing a few industrial sites along the way. Beyond Pepper St., the trail gets noticeably less use and weeds have encroached at the edges of the prepared surface. It slips between a few ledge outcroppings, crosses a private road, and then ends at the Newtown town line.

BACKGROUND:

The trail follows the course of the Housatonic Railroad, one of New England's first railroads which made its maiden run to Monroe in 1840. Operating passenger and freight service to Bridgeport, the line was acquired in the early 1890's by the New York, New Haven, and Hartford Railroad but began to struggle in the mid-1900's when automobile and truck transportation took hold. Use of the line ceased in 1962 and the rails and ties were removed.

Local residents eventually urged the town to acquire the corridor for use as a trail and in the mid-1990's the town secured a federal grant for its development. The rail-trail opened for use in 1999 and its expansion has been proposed in two directions: northward to Botsford Station in Newtown and southward to connect Trumbull's segment of the route (Chapter 2) and eventually to Bridgeport.

The trail links Wolfe Park, a town-owned recreation area, where 300-plus acres offer swimming facilities, picnic areas, walking trails, and athletic fields. An admission fee is charged.

DRIVING DIRECTIONS:

From Rte. 15 (Merritt Pkwy.), take Exit 49 and follow Rte. 25 north. Where the divided highway ends, continue on Rte. 25 north for 3 miles to the village of Upper Stepney, then turn right on Pepper St. Continue for 1 mile, turn right on Cutler's Farm Rd., then immediately left at the parking lot.

TOILETS:

Wolfe Park at Great Hollow Lake

ADDITIONAL INFORMATION:

Monroe Parks and Recreation Dept., (203) 452-5416

4 Shelton Lakes Recreation Path

Shelton, CT

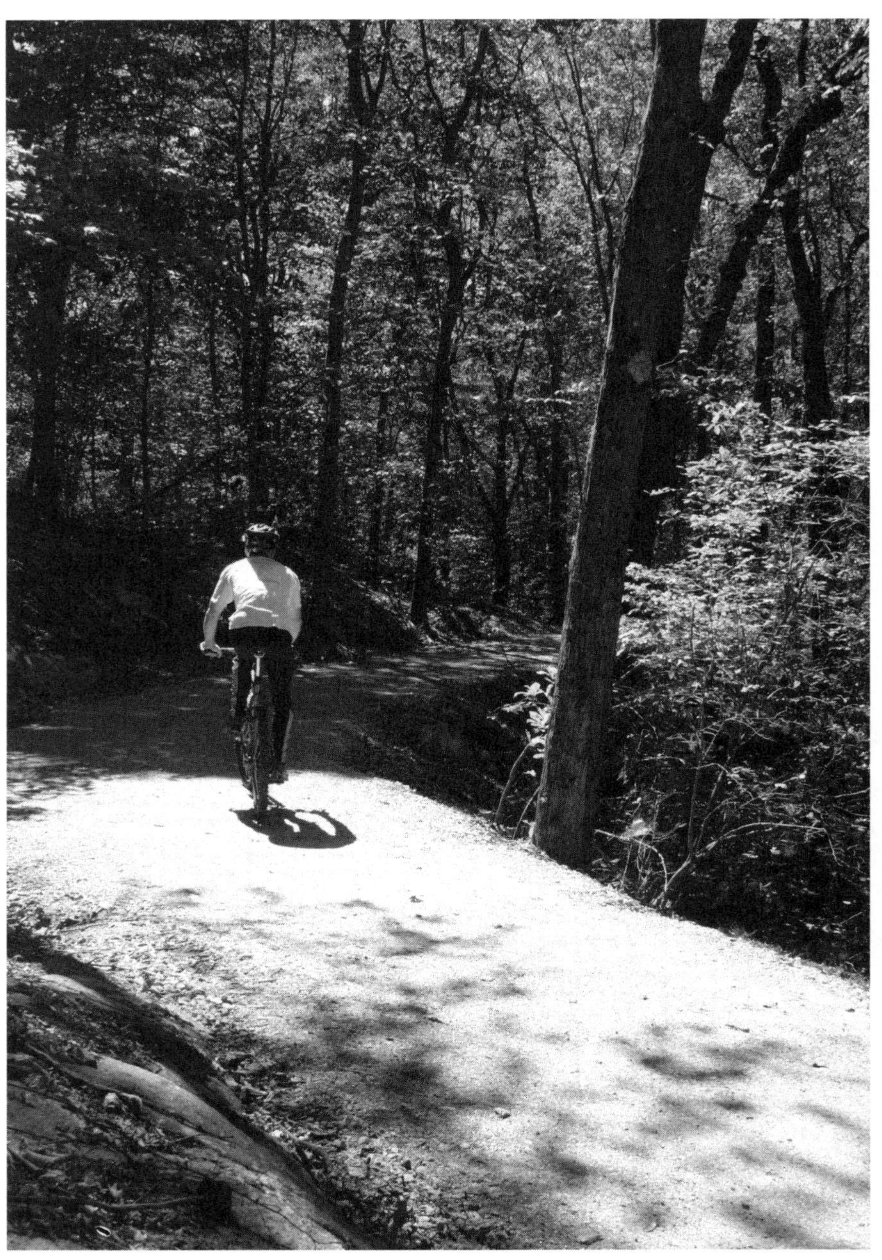

LENGTH: 4.3 miles
SURFACE: processed stone (except unfinished midsection)
TERRAIN: hilly
NOTE: quarter-mile-long unfinished midsection is rough

A hilly alternative, this woodsy recreation path has a firm surface and a curvy route through a natural landscape of ponds, streams, and huge ledge outcroppings.

RULES & SAFETY:

• Bicyclists should yield to pedestrians.

• This especially hilly and curvy trail deserves caution. Keep to the right, ride at a safe speed, and alert others (*"On our left..."*) when approaching from behind.

• Be especially cautious in the presence of children and pets, since their movements can be unpredictable.

• Dogs must be leashed and their wastes removed.

ORIENTATION:

Yellow blazes mark the trail and crosswalks guide it across roads. The processed stone surface is wide and firm although the material varies and some sections are smoother than others. A quarter-mile segment of the trail south of Oak Valley Rd. remains in development and, as a result, requires either mountain biking skills or walking until the surfacing is completed.

The trail encounters relatively big hills. Its highest elevation is near the midsection at the powerlines and the lowest elevation is the Pine Lake trailhead, the recommended starting point. Limited parking is available at Constitution Blvd. but none is provided at the Lane St. end.

TRAIL DESCRIPTION:

The Recreation Path begins at a bridge over the outlet stream at **Pine Lake**. Circling the north shore in a pine forest, it rises on a short hill and descends the other side before reaching **Meadow St.** (0.3 miles).

Here a three-quarter-mile uphill slope begins, first with a paved surface for the 0.3 miles to school playing fields and then with a crushed stone surface. Crossing **Constitution**

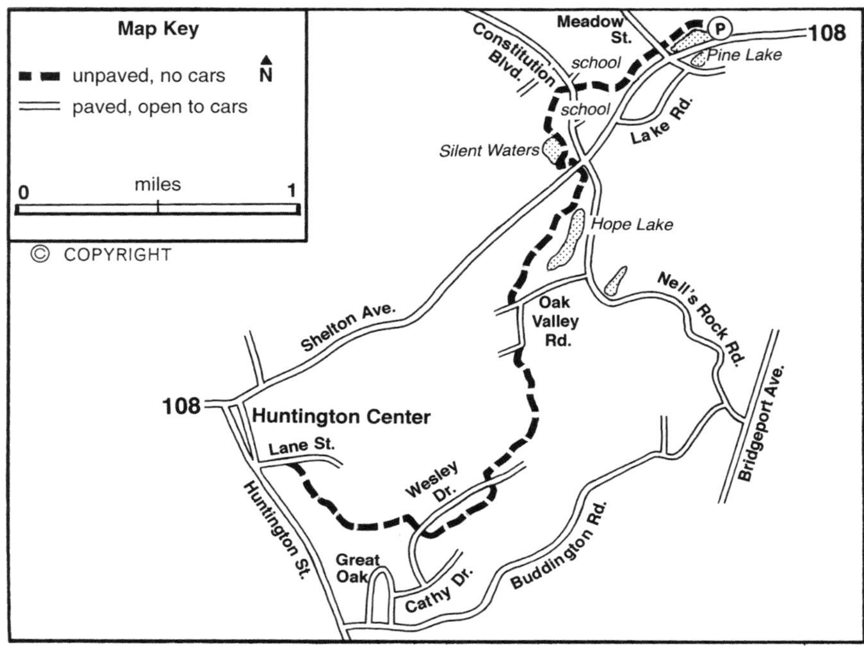

Blvd. (0.8 miles), the trail climbs until the 1-mile mark where it turns abruptly left on a long empoundment dam at **Silent Waters** and circles the eastern shore. Ahead, a wooden bridge over the spillway offers a view over the pond.

After another sharp left turn at the end of the dam, the trail drops to the intersection of **Rte. 108** and **Nell's Rock Rd.** (1.4 miles) at a crosswalk and signal. It returns to woods on the other side and climbs for another third of a mile, first with a strenuous slope to the dam at **Hope Lake** and then with an easier grade. Flattening at the top, it winds past stone walls, ledge outcroppings, and mountain laurel bushes before emerging at a set of powerlines (2 miles).

Just ahead, the trail passes a metal gate and turns left along a private driveway to emerge at **Oak Valley Rd.** (2.2 miles). Turn right (south) and follow the pavement along the powerlines for 0.2 miles to the end, then keep right on a private drive and look for the trail forking left at another metal gate. Although it is due for improvement, the trail's next quarter-mile has no prepared surface and the rough conditions require either mountain biking skills or walking.

The prepared surface resumes at 2.6 miles where the trail veers right (west) from the powerline corridor and descends into woods. The next half-mile ranks among the prettiest as the trail curves between wetlands and rock outcroppings, but several sharp corners deserve caution. After crossing **Wesley Dr.** (3.2 miles) at a residential neighborhood, the trail enjoys a downhill slope for a half-mile to a second crossing of Wesley Dr. where it drops abruptly onto the roadway.

It climbs briefly on the other side past several homes, then curves downhill through woods to the 4-mile mark at a large field. The trail skirts the edge and soon ends at **Lane St.** (4.3 miles) near the village of **Huntington Center**.

BACKGROUND:

A strong community effort created this trail. Utilizing grants, town-owned lands, generously low construction bids, and the efforts of both town staff and volunteer citizens, Shelton's Conservation Commission has built this ambitious trail at an affordable price over the span of only a few years. The trail remains a work in progress but is nearly complete.

DRIVING DIRECTIONS:

Rte. 8 southbound: Take Exit 14. Follow Rte. 110 north for 0.4 miles, turn left on Rte. 108 south, and follow it for 1 mile to the Pine Lake trailhead parking lot on the right.

Rte. 8 northbound: Take Exit 15. Follow Rte. 34 west for 0.4 miles to a traffic signal, turn left on Bridge St. and cross the river, turn left on Rte. 110 south, then right on Rte. 108 south. Follow Rte. 108 for 1 mile to the Pine Lake parking lot on the right.

Rte. 15 southbound: Take Exit 58. Follow Rte. 34 west for 3.5 miles to a traffic signal, turn left on Bridge St. and cross the river, then as above.

TOILETS:

none provided

ADDITIONAL INFORMATION:

www.sheltonconservation.org/recreation/shelton_trails.html

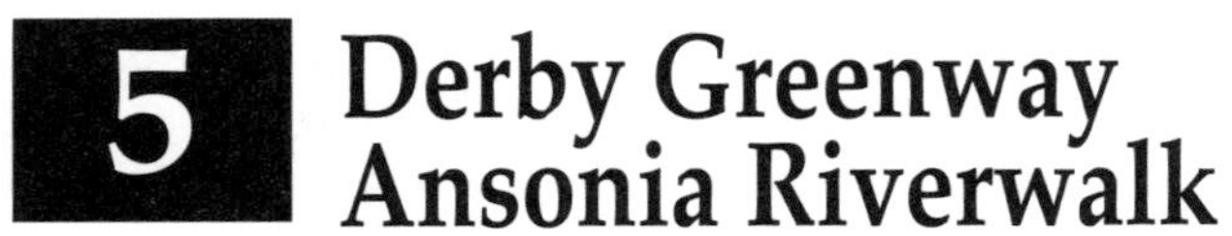

5 Derby Greenway Ansonia Riverwalk

Derby - Ansonia, CT

LENGTH: 2.3 miles
SURFACE: paved
TERRAIN: short slopes

Overlooking the confluence of the Naugatuck and the Housatonic rivers, these short trails thread a precise course along riverbanks, railroads, and roadways to form a useful greenway close to downtown Derby. Tree cover is scarce so it's exposed to wind and hot summer sun.

RULES & SAFETY:

- Bicyclists should yield to pedestrians.
- The trail is curvy and has a speed limit of 8 m.p.h.
- Use extra caution in crowded areas and when children and pets are present, since their movements can be unpredictable.
- Keep to the right, pass on the left, and alert others (*"On your left..."*) when approaching from behind.
- Help keep it clean by carrying out all that you carry in.
- Dogs must be leashed and their wastes removed.
- The greenway is open from sunrise to sunset.

ORIENTATION:

These greenways join to form a continuous trail in the neighboring cities of Derby and Ansonia. The trail is confined to a narrow space along two rivers, two railroads, and a highway, and access points include two trailheads. The most popular starting point is at the city line on Division St. where the Derby Greenway extends southward and the Ansonia Riverwalk extends northward. Parking is provided on both sides of Division St. and a crosswalk joins the two.

An ample supply of benches is provided beside the trail along with protective fencing, landscaping, and mileage markers. Most of the trail follows the top of flood control embankments along the rivers, so water views are abundant but trees and shade are limited to the trail's southernmost point in the area known as O'Sullivan's Island at the confluence of the rivers. As a result, much of the trail is exposed to both wind and hot summer sun.

TRAIL DESCRIPTION:

Begin at the **Division St.** trailhead where two parking lots and a landscaped setting provide a welcoming gateway for the trail near a busy retail area. Running northward, the **Ansonia Riverwalk** heads upstream beside the **Naugatuck River** for just over a half-mile along the flat top of a floodwall embankment, built to protect the city during periods of high water. Wood fencing corrals the trail along this high vantage point which offers views across the river to downtown Ansonia. After curving past a sewage treatment plant, the trail's pavement ends before reaching an active railroad.

To the south, the **Derby Greenway** runs for 1.7 miles. It begins on the same flat floodwall for the first 0.8 miles heading downstream on the Naugatuck, with fencing protecting both sides of the trail from the embankment's big slopes. At **Rte. 34**, the trail turns and descends in tight switchbacks in order to pass underneath the roadway, with another fence separating railroad tracks at the bottom near the Derby **train station**.

Emerging on the other side, the trail continues southward until just past the 1-mile mark where it turns sharply right (west), passes under the railroad, and reaches a T-intersection. Turning left, a short spur currently dead ends at several benches overlooking the river but planned construction will extend this trail. Turning right, the trail continues into the tree cover and green surroundings of **O'Sullivan's Island** and circles a small pond in a landscaped setting of mowed grass and more benches.

A short distance ahead, the trail reaches a second T-intersection. Straight ahead, a spur leads to a boat launch on the **Housatonic River**. To the right (north), the main trail

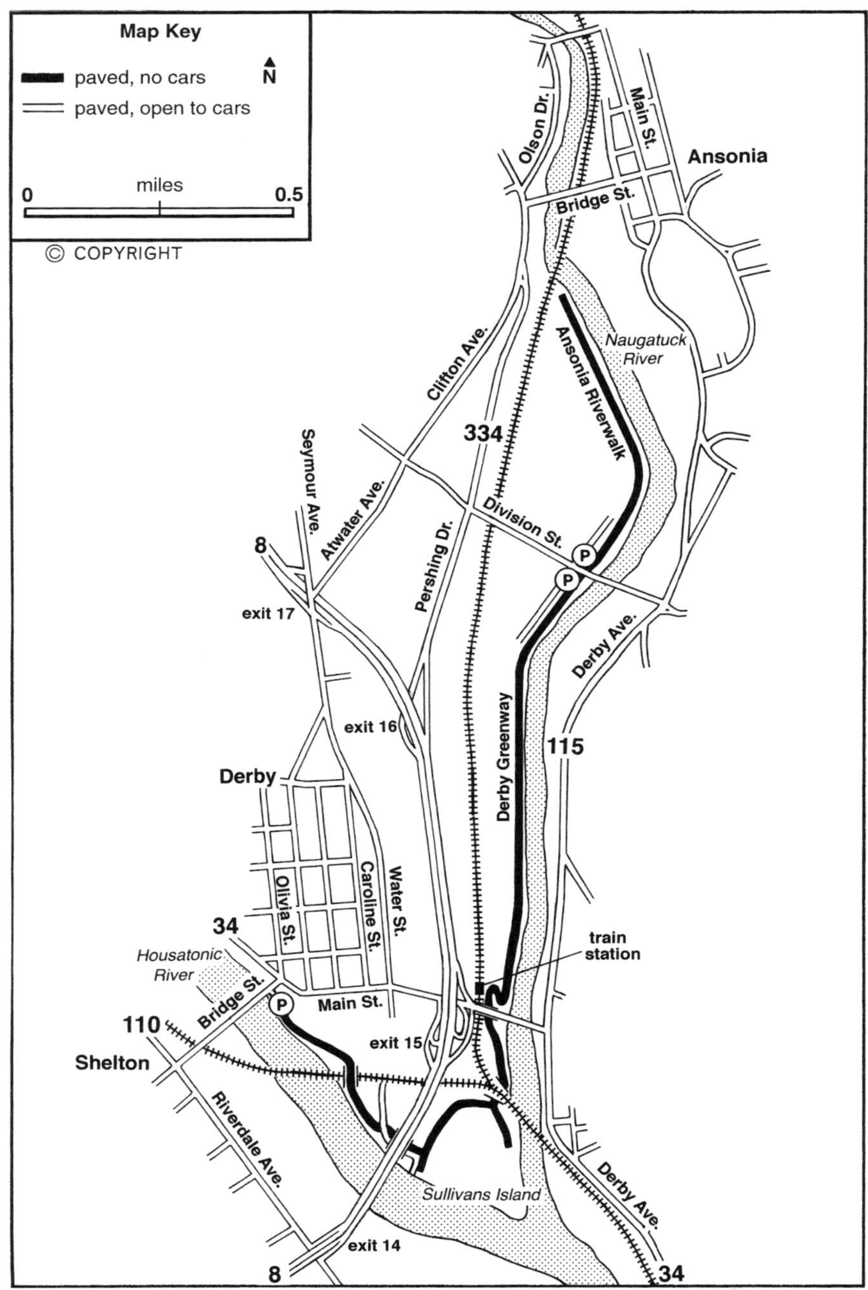
Map Key
paved, no cars
paved, open to cars
N
0
miles
0.5
© COPYRIGHT
Olson Dr.
Main St.
Ansonia
Bridge St.
Clifton Ave.
Ansonia Riverwalk
Naugatuck River
334
Seymour Ave.
Atwater Ave.
Division St.
8
Pershing Dr.
P
P
exit 17
Derby Ave.
exit 16
Derby Greenway
115
Derby
Olivia St.
Caroline St.
Water St.
34
Housatonic River
train station
Bridge St.
P
Main St.
110
exit 15
Shelton
Riverdale Ave.
Sullivans Island
Derby Ave.
exit 14
8
34

rises on an abrupt slope, passes underneath a highway bridge for **Rte. 8**, then joins the boat launch access road for a short distance. The trail separates on the other side of this road and rises to a high bicycle/pedestrian bridge over another railroad with a broad view of the Housatonic and downtown Shelton on the other side. After descending the bridge, the trail continues upstream along the Housatonic on the crest of another flood control embankment with wood fencing guiding the trail to its terminus at the **Bridge St.** trailhead parking area.

BACKGROUND:

The Derby Greenway opened in 2006 and the Ansonia Riverwalk opened in 2011. Both trails were created using federal transportation funds and local matching funds in an effort to reclaim underused areas as public greenspace, create alternative means of transportation, and to inspire people to exercise. They are the first steps toward a regional trail effort known as the Naugatuck Valley Greenway.

Future trail construction is planned or proposed in numerous directions. Derby is poised to expand the Greenway at O'Sullivan's Island by completing a loop off the existing trail. Ansonia will extend the Riverwalk northward over the railroad and across the Naugatuck River. Other proposed linkages will reach Shelton and Orange.

DRIVING DIRECTIONS:

Rte. 8 northbound: Take Exit 16 for Pershing Dr. Continue for a third of a mile, turn right on Division St., and drive for 0.2 miles to a traffic signal and intersection at the crossing of the trail, just before a bridge over the river. Turn either left or right for trailhead parking lots.

Rte. 8 southbound: Take Exit 18. Turn left on Seymour Ave., then immediately right on Atwater Ave. and drive for a third of a mile. Turn right on Division St. and continue for 0.4 miles to a traffic signal and intersection at the trail crossing, just before a bridge over the river. Turn either left or right for trailhead parking lots.

TOILETS:

none provided

ADDITIONAL INFORMATION:

www.cogcnv.org/greenway/

6 Larkin State Park Trail

Naugatuck - Southbury, CT

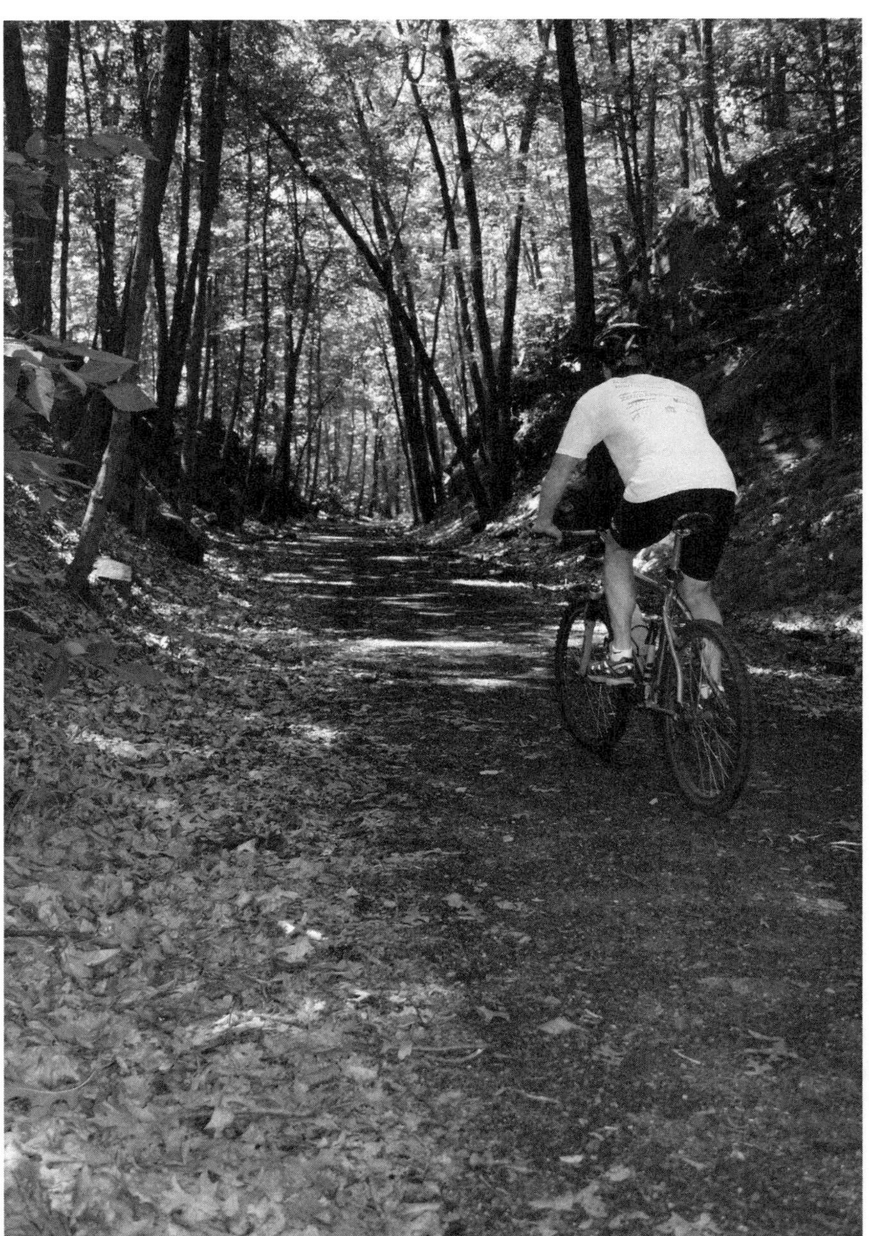

LENGTH: 10.7 miles
SURFACE: gravel
TERRAIN: gentle slopes
NOTE: wide-tired bicycles recommended

A former railroad, the Larkin State Park Trail tames a forested terrain of hills and wetlands with an even grade for bicycling, walking, and horseback riding. Several rough spots make wide-tired bicycles preferable.

RULES & SAFETY:

• Bicyclists should yield to pedestrians and horseback riders.

• Ride at a safe speed, keep to the right side, and alert others (*"On your left..."*) when approaching from behind.

• Stop at road intersections and assume that drivers do not see you.

• Use extra caution when horses are present since they can be unfamiliar with bicycles and prone to panic. Make verbal contact with the rider well in advance so that the animal will feel safe, and be ready to stop at the side of the trail if necessary.

• Wear blaze orange clothing if possible during hunting season in the late fall.

• Be careful not to block trailhead gates when parking since work crews and emergency vehicles need access.

• Much of the trail is remote so be self-sufficient with food, water, and bicycle repair supplies.

• Motorized vehicles are prohibited.

• The trail is open from sunrise to sunset.

ORIENTATION:

The Larkin State Park Trail is aligned in a mostly east-west direction with a designated parking lot located at the eastern terminus on Rte. 63 in Naugatuck. Minimal parking space is available at other trail/road intersections including Strongtown Rd. (Rte. 188) in Southbury, Christian St. in Oxford, and Towantic Hill Rd. in Oxford south of Towantic Pond.

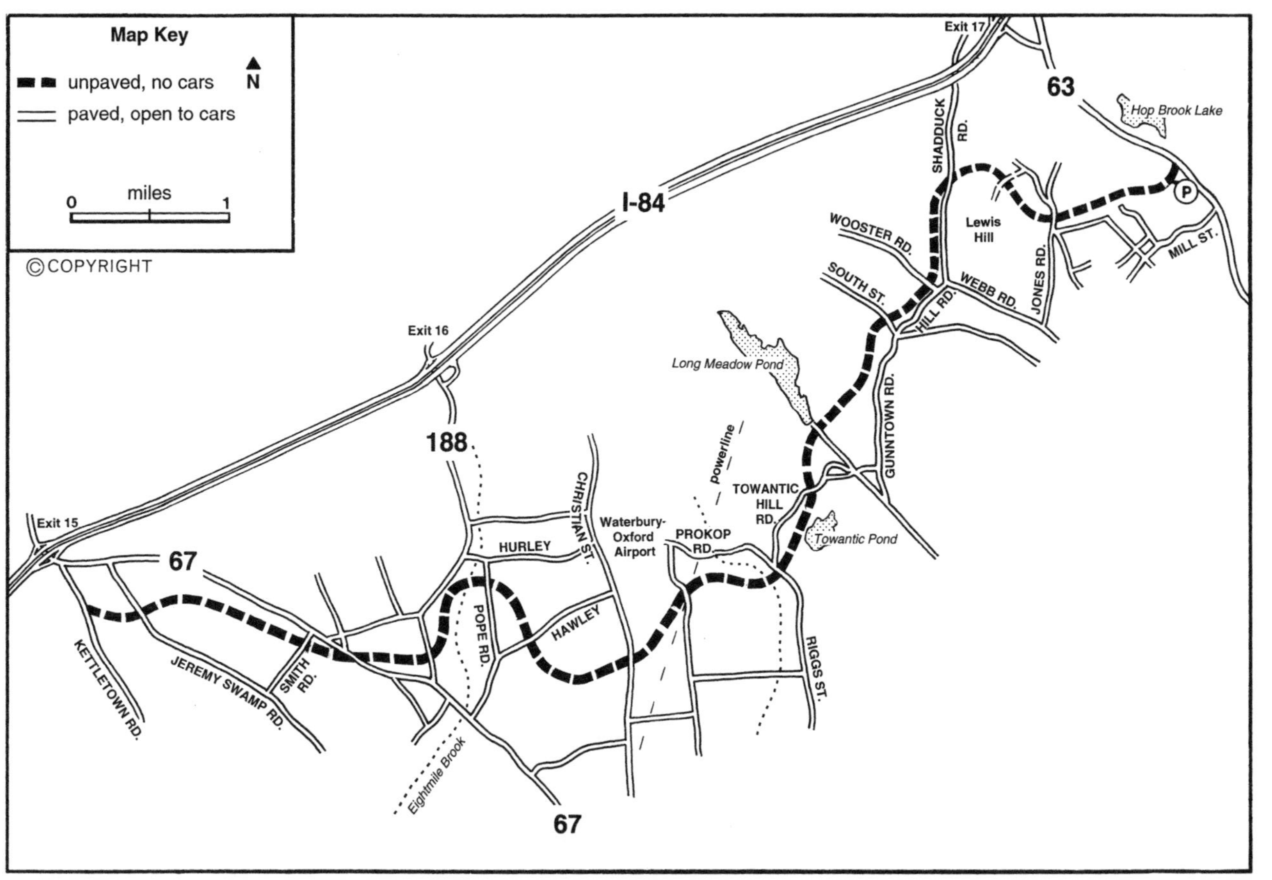
Map Key
unpaved, no cars
paved, open to cars
N
miles
0
1
©COPYRIGHT
Exit 17
63
Hop Brook Lake
I-84
SHADDUCK RD.
Lewis Hill
WOOSTER RD.
SOUTH ST.
HILL RD.
WEBB RD.
JONES RD.
MILL ST.
Exit 16
Long Meadow Pond
GUNNTOWN RD.
188
powerline
TOWANTIC HILL RD.
Towantic Pond
CHRISTIAN ST.
Waterbury-Oxford Airport
PROKOP RD.
Exit 15
HURLEY
67
POPE RD.
HAWLEY
RIGGS ST.
KETTLETOWN RD.
JEREMY SWAMP RD.
SMITH RD.
Eightmile Brook
67

The highest elevation along the trail's 10.7-mile route is the midpoint between Towantic Hill Rd. and Christian St. with gentle slopes declining toward each end.

Most of the trail has a smooth, hard-packed surface but a few areas have exposed rocks, horse hoof prints, or brief detours from the rail bed at road crossings which hold rougher conditions. In general, surface conditions are smoothest along the eastern end and midsection of the trail, and most difficult along parts of the western end especially in the vicinity of Rte. 67 in Southbury.

The trail remains in a relatively undeveloped, simple state. Crosswalks and signs do not exist at road crossings so use appropriate caution when crossing roads and assume that drivers do not see you. Although road intersections are numerous, much of the trail is remote so be prepared with adequate food, water, and repair supplies.

TRAIL DESCRIPTION:

From the trailhead on **Rte. 63** in Naugatuck, take the curving path uphill through the woods to the rail bed, reached in a short distance. Turn left and follow the firm, smooth surface westward through woods on a slight uphill grade, first as it slices through an outcropping of ledge and then as it passes a few housing developments on the left.

The incline lasts for about a mile with an interruption at an abrupt drop to **Jones Rd.** at the site of a missing bridge. The trail travels high above the surrounding forest floor on elevated grades which bridge low-lying areas, then flattens as it hugs the side of **Lewis Hill** and circles its northern slope.

Crossing **Shadduck Rd.** after the 2-mile mark, the trail turns southward into Middlebury and tilts upward again on another incline which lasts for the next 2 miles. It cuts through more bedrock as it parallels **Shadduck Rd.**, then intersects **Wooster Rd.** (2.6 miles) and **South St.** (3.0 miles) at the site of a missing bridge.

The trail clings to the sides of hills and uses earthen causeways to bridge low spots in between before emerging at a small settlement of houses on **Griswold Rd.** (3.9 miles) near the southern end of **Long Meadow Pond**, where it enters Oxford. The pond is barely visible behind a dam.

Just ahead, the trail intersects **Towantic Hill Rd.** (4.3 miles) at a former bridge site which has been filled. Watch for a path detouring on the left side and follow it up a banking to cross the pavement.

Reaching the trail's highest elevation, the next 1.9 miles have a flatter profile and a mowed border of grass for much of the way. The trail enters a more open environment near **Towantic Pond** and passes its boggy, western shoreline with a half-mile straightaway, then intersects Towantic Hill Rd. (4.9 miles) again. Curving westward for a short distance, it skirts wetlands along **Jacks Brook** and then passes under a **powerline** near the intersection of **Larkey Rd.** (5.6 miles). Along the next half-mile, note that low-flying aircraft are frequently seen approaching nearby **Waterbury-Oxford Airport**.

Christian St. (6.2 miles) marks the start of a slight downhill grade which lasts for the remaining 4.5 miles. The trail crosses another causeway built over a wetland, turns northward, and makes a short detour off the rail bed at the intersection of **Hawley Rd.** (7.0 miles). After returning to the rail bed on the other side, the trail reverses its course with a 180-degree turn back to the south, crossing **Pope Rd.** (7.5 miles) and a causeway over **Eightmile Brook** along the way.

Entering Southbury, it curves back to the west at the crossing of **Rte. 188** (**Strongtown Rd.**) near the 8.3-mile mark. Surface conditions along the next half-mile deteriorate with a narrowing treadway from encroaching foliage, drainage problems where the trail passes through a cut in the hillside, and a rough detour at the intersection of busy **Rte. 67** (8.8 miles). After crossing the road, follow the driveway downhill to the right and look for the rail-trail ahead on the right side.

The downhill grade is more pronounced at this point and suffers from more drainage problems for a short distance. The trail joins a driveway on the way to **Smith Rd.** (9.2 miles), then crosses the street and follows a straight, smooth line for the next half-mile. A final detour is required at a missing bridge over **Jeremy Swamp Rd.** (10.3 miles) where a footpath drops down an embankment and climbs back to the rail bed on the other side. The last stretch to **Kettletown Rd.** (10.7 miles) offers easy rolling over flat ground with a grassy surface.

BACKGROUND:

The New York and New England Railroad completed this route between western Connecticut and New York in 1881 using the manual labor of Irish immigrants. Following the railroad's bankruptcy in 1894, the line became part of the New York, New Haven, and Hartford and provided freight and passenger service into the 1930's, when it ceased operations.

Charles L. Larkin saw the value of the abandoned rail bed as a linear park and gifted it to the state for use as a bridle trail in 1943. Other segments of this rail line have also become bike paths, including the Hop River State Park Trail (Chapter 30) and the Washington Secondary Bike Path/Moosup Valley State Park Trail (Chapter 37).

DRIVING DIRECTIONS:

From I-84 westbound: Take Exit 17 and follow signs for Rte. 64 west. Turn left on Rte. 63 south and continue for 2.8 miles to the parking lot on the right.

From I-84 eastbound: Take Exit 17 and turn right on Rte. 63 south. Drive for 2.1 miles to the parking lot on the right.

From Rte. 8: Take Exit 26 and follow Rte. 63 north for 2.5 miles to the parking lot on the left.

TOILETS:

none on site

ADDITIONAL INFORMATION:

Larkin State Park Trail, c/o Southford Falls State Park, Quaker Farms Rd., Southbury, CT 06488, Tel. (203) 264-5169

7 Middlebury Greenway

Middlebury, CT

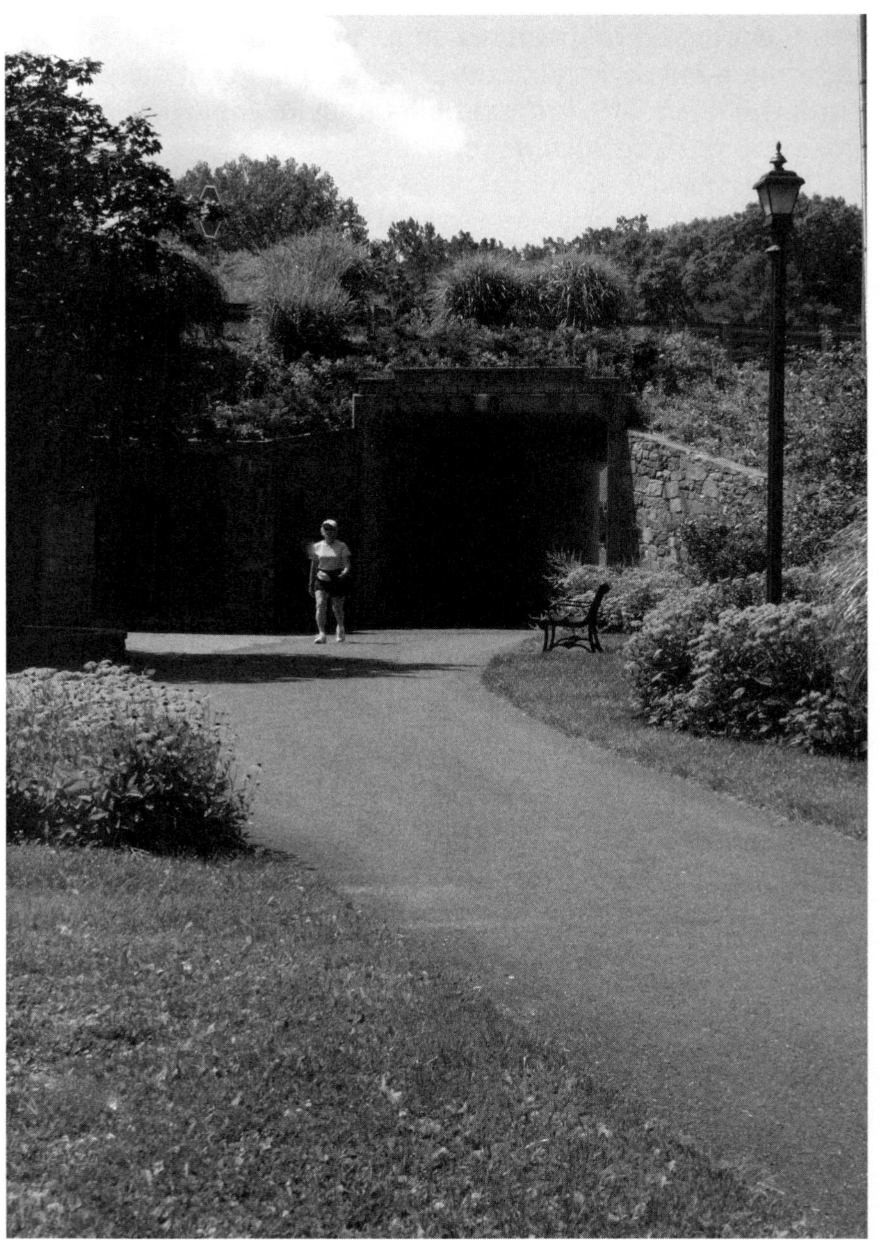

LENGTH: 4.7 miles
SURFACE: paved
TERRAIN: hilly

Spanning the town along a former trolley line, this rolling, landscaped trail is an attractive option for walkers, runners, and bicyclists eager to avoid nearby traffic.

RULES & SAFETY:

- Bicyclists should yield to pedestrians.
- Keep to the right, pass on the left, and alert others (*"On your left..."*) when approaching from behind.
- The trail is hilly and curvy. Ride at a safe speed and use extra caution when children and pets are present.
- In-line skating and skateboarding are not permitted.
- Move off the trail when stopped so others can pass.
- Dogs must be leashed and their wastes removed.
- A sign at the trailhead reads: *Take only photographs, leave only footprints, keep only memories.*

ORIENTATION:

The greenway parallels Rte. 64 in roughly the east-west direction between Lake Quassapaug and Rte. 63. Where space is limited, a few short sections do not have a separated pathway and instead follow roads, but traffic at these points is minimal. Two trailhead parking lots provide access along the trail, with additional parking available at Meadowview Park. Elevation varies, with the highest point being near the western trailhead and the lowest point being near the eastern trailhead.

The greenway is generously equipped with fencing along steep bankings, barricades to prevent vehicle entry, and crosswalks at road intersections. In addition, attractive landscaping adorns the route with plantings, grass borders, and benches.

TRAIL DESCRIPTION:

Starting at the western trailhead parking lot beside **Rte. 64**, the greenway heads in two directions. To the west, it lasts for only a third of a mile with a descent to a playing

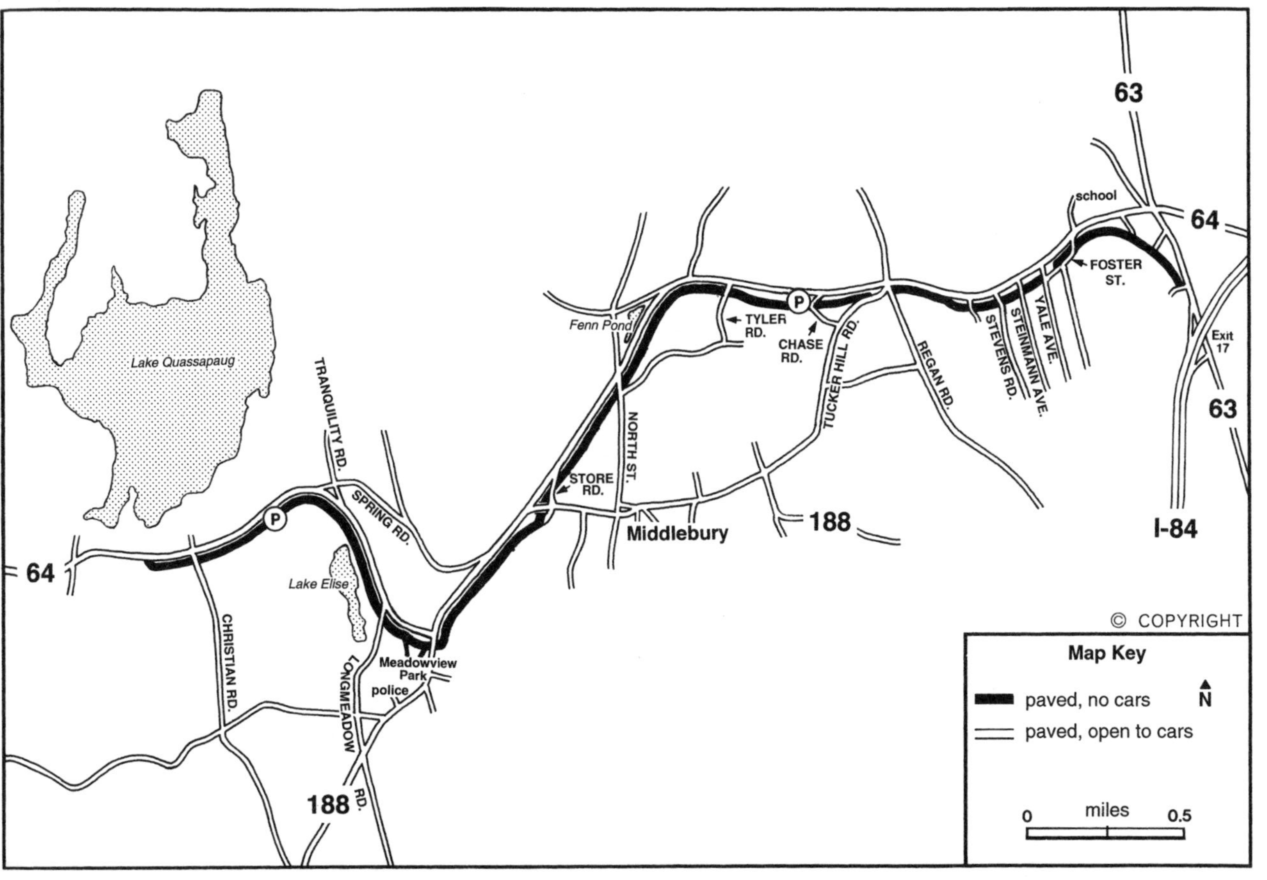

63
school
64
FOSTER ST.
Exit 17
63
I-84
STEVENS RD.
STEINMANN AVE.
YALE AVE.
REGAN RD.
TUCKER HILL RD.
P
TYLER RD.
CHASE RD.
Fenn Pond
NORTH ST.
STORE RD.
Middlebury
188
Lake Quassapaug
TRANQUILITY RD.
SPRING RD.
P
64
Lake Elise
CHRISTIAN RD.
LONGMEADOW RD.
Meadowview Park
police
188
© COPYRIGHT
Map Key
paved, no cars
paved, open to cars
N
0
miles
0.5

field across from **Lake Quassapaug** and the Quassy Amusement Park, a popular summer attraction. To the east, the trail runs for 4.5 miles with mostly downhill pedaling to **Rte. 63**.

Riding eastward, bicyclists pass caution signs warning of an impending downhill curve. The pavement tilts downward for a third of a mile on a moderate slope with a right-hand bend, crossing a few driveways near the bottom where riders must maneuver through barricade posts. Halfway down this hill at the intersection of **Tranquility Rd.** and **Spring Rd.** (across Rte. 64) notice a stone shelter which once served as a trolley stop.

At the bottom, the slope reverses to a slight incline where a row of utility poles stands in the path near **Lake Elise**. The trail crosses **Longmeadow Rd.** (0.7 miles) at the top of the rise and then curves back to the left on a slope above the playing fields of **Meadowview Park**. It then descends with a few curves to the park's small playground and parking lot and crosses **Rte. 188** at a traffic signal about a mile from the western trailhead parking lot.

Here a 0.4-mile incline begins. Turning left and following the edge of Rte. 188 and Rte. 64, the trail climbs a moderate slope in a landscaped area of shrubs, fencing, and a few benches, then veers from the road at the top and descends along a powerline to a small parking lot.

It continues into a tunnel under Rte. 188 (1.6 miles) near the center of Middlebury. After exiting on the other side, notice another trolley stop built into the wall on the right at a circle of benches. The trail coasts downhill for another tenth of a mile beside a wooden fence and **Store Rd.**, then crosses and continues downward. A strip of trees and a banking provide extra separation from parallel Rte. 64 along the next third of a mile to **North St.**, where the trail returns to the edge of the road.

Reaching a temporary stretch of level ground across from **Fenn Pond**, the trail crosses a wooden bridge over Goat Brook, then bends to the right and crosses **Tyler Rd.**

(2.7 miles) at the start of another gradual descent. The next quarter-mile to the trailhead parking lot at **Chase Rd.** is screened from the traffic by another tree-covered banking and enjoys the sight of Goat Brook as it tumbles downhill.

Continuing eastward, the downward run lasts for another quarter-mile to **Tucker Hill Rd.** (3.2 miles) at a low point near Hop Brook, passing through a cut in the bedrock of a small hill along the way. The greenway follows a sidewalk along Rte. 64 for a short distance before separating from the roadway and descending across **Stevens Rd.** (3.7 miles) to Long Swamp Brook.

Here a cluster of road intersections deserves caution. Crossing **Steinmann Ave.**, the greenway climbs steeply to **Yale Ave.**, crosses the road and follows **Foster St.** for a short distance, then resumes with a separated pathway on the left. After crossing Foster St. again, the trail rounds a corner on a slope above Rte. 64 and then coasts down to the side of **Rte. 63** near Exit 17 of **I-84**, 4.4 miles from the western trailhead.

BACKGROUND:

The greenway follows the rail bed of a former trolley line which ran from the city of Waterbury to Middlebury and Woodbury. Opened in 1908 by the Connecticut Company, the trolley provided a major improvement for commerce and transportation in the area by allowing Middlebury's residents easy access to the city and Waterbury's population an enjoyable way to visit the countryside.

In the warm season, the company offered open-air cars which brought crowds of visitors from Waterbury to Lake Quassapaug, a summer retreat in Middlebury. The ticket price was 15 cents.

The popularity of automobiles and buses forced the closing of the trolley line in 1930 and the tracks were quickly removed for scrap metal. After lingering for about 60 years, the route was reborn in 1992 as a multi-use trail stretching for 3.3 miles from Lake Quassapaug to Chase Rd. Additional construction in subsequent years has extended it eastward for another 1.5 miles to Rte. 63.

DRIVING DIRECTIONS:

western trailhead parking lot: From I-84, take Exit 16 and follow Rte. 188 north for 2.7 miles. Turn left on Rte. 64 west and continue for 1 mile to the parking lot on the left at the top of a hill. (If you pass the Quassy Amusement Park, you have gone too far.)

Chase Rd. trailhead parking lot: From I-84 take Exit 17 and follow signs for Rte. 64 west. From the intersection of Rte. 63, drive for 1.3 miles on Rte. 64 west and turn left on Chase Rd. Park in the lot immediately on the right.

TOILETS:

police station at Meadowview Park

ADDITIONAL INFORMATION:

Middlebury Parks & Recreation Dept., Tel. (202) 758-2520, www.middlebury-ct.org/Pages/ParksandRecreation.aspx

8 Railroad Ramble

Salisbury, CT

LENGTH: 2.1 miles
SURFACE: mowed grass, dirt
TERRAIN: flat

Tucked in the beautiful hills of Connecticut's northwest corner, Salisbury's quiet rail-trail resembles a green carpet stretched between the town's two village centers.

RULES & SAFETY:

- Bicyclists yield to pedestrians and horses.
- Ride at a safe speed and use extra caution when children and pets are present.
- Alert others (*"On your left..."*) when approaching from behind to avoid startling them.
- Respect the private property along the trail.

ORIENTATION:

The trail parallels Rte. 44 between the village centers of Salisbury and Lakeville. Although relatively undeveloped, it has a mowed grass surface for most of the way, gates or barricades at road crossings, and a few informational signs. No trailhead parking lot exists so visitors are advised to park beside Library St. near the trail's northern terminus.

TRAIL DESCRIPTION:

Heading north from **Library St.**, the trail lasts for only a half-mile, beginning on the pavement of **Railroad St.** and then continuing into woods at a gate on the left with a gravel surface. After passing a few homes, it merges with a gravel driveway before reaching **E. Main St.** (**Rte. 44**).

Heading south from Library St., the trail extends for 1.6 miles through mostly open surroundings of fields and wetlands. It starts following the edge of a field with a view, crosses **Salmon Kill Rd.**, then turns southwest and enters a scenic area of ponds, brooks, and wetlands on a three-

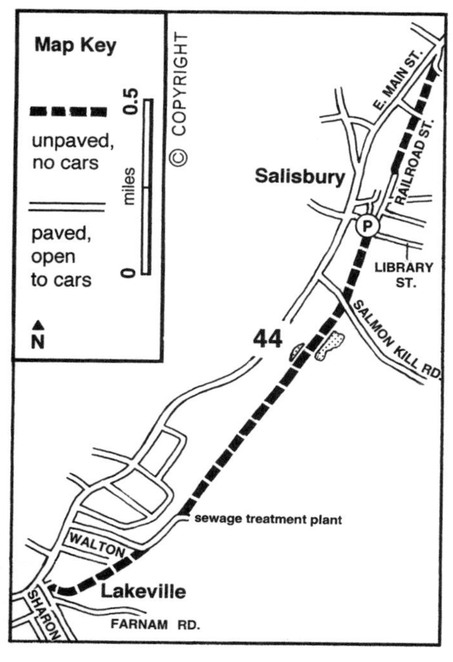

quarter-mile straight-line course.

A mile south of Library St., the trail passes Salisbury's **sewage treatment plant** and follows its paved access road for a quarter-mile. Where the pavement turns right at the end of **Walton Rd.**, the trail continues straight on a narrow width of mowed grass with thick foliage along the sides.

The trail approaches **Lakeville** on an elevated grade beside a ballfield. Before reaching the site of a missing bridge over **Farnam Rd.** and Factory Brook, it descends the west side of the embankment along a fence to the edge of the field and then ends at **Sharon Rd.**

BACKGROUND:

Originally called the Connecticut Western, this railroad stretched from Collinsville to Millerton, NY in 1871 linking Hartford with Poughkeepsie. Following construction of a bridge across the Hudson River in 1888, it became one of the dominant rail lines between New England and New York.

Trucks and interstate highways eventually prevailed, and the last train rolled down the tracks in 1965. Soon after, the town acquired this 2-mile section of the route for use as a trail.

DRIVING DIRECTIONS:

Salisbury is located on Rte. 44 approximately 51 miles west of I-84 in Hartford and 25 miles west of Rte. 8 in Winsted. Turn left on Library St. in downtown Salisbury beside the stone library and continue around the first hard right turn, then park beside the road.

TOILETS:

library, when it's open

9 Sue Grossman Still River Greenway

Torrington-Winchester, CT

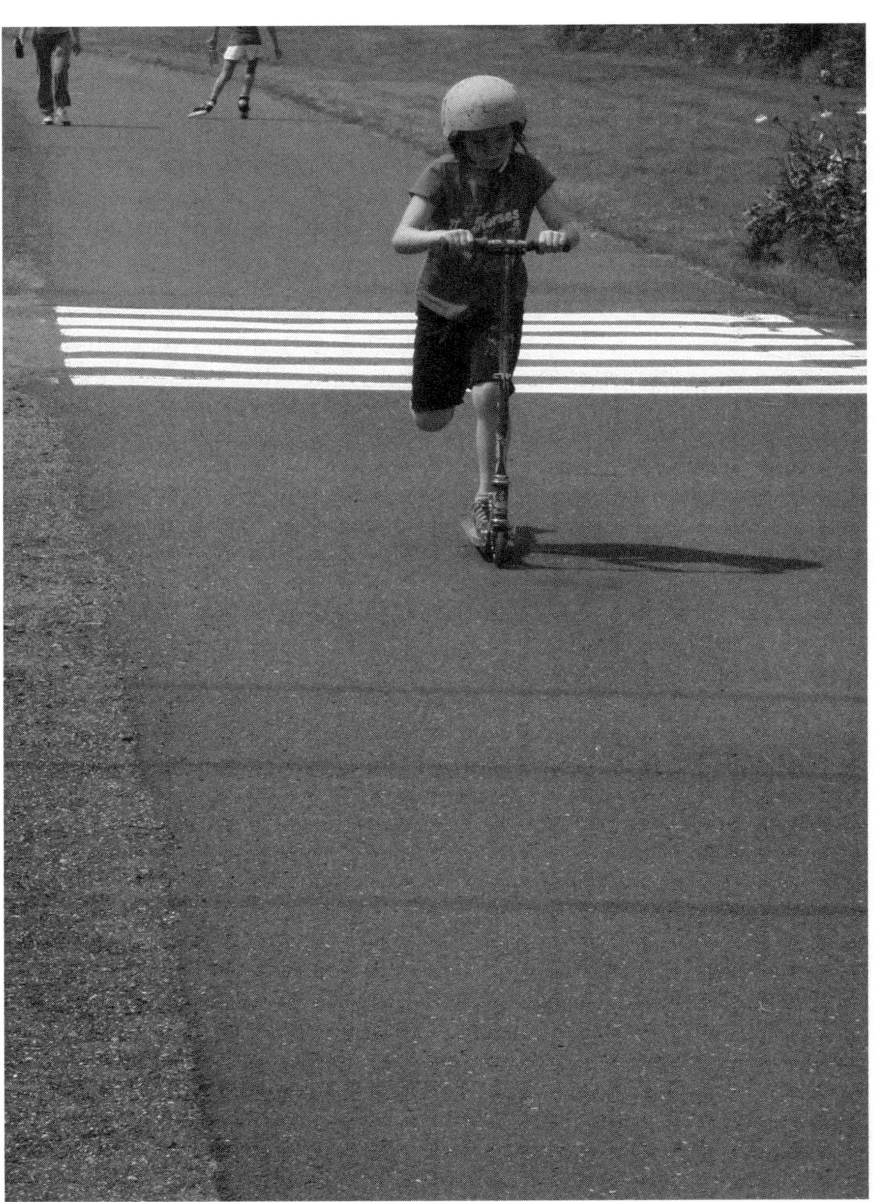

LENGTH: 2.8 miles
SURFACE: paved
TERRAIN: flat

Road noise is often close but this well-kept rail-trail provides welcome exercise space and peaceful scenery along the Still River. Little shade exists on the trail so be prepared during hot weather.

RULES & SAFETY:

- Bicyclists should yield to pedestrians.
- Keep to the right, pass on the left, and alert others (*"On your left..."*) when approaching from behind.
- Ride at a safe speed, and use extra caution when children and pets are present.
- Dogs must be leashed and their wastes removed.
- The greenway is open from dawn until dusk.

ORIENTATION:

The trail has a north-south alignment and parallels Winsted Rd. for its entire length from Harris Rd. in Torrington to Lanson Rd. in Winchester. Intersecting streets serve as useful landmarks along the way. Crosswalks and signage are present, wooden fencing borders the trail where necessary, and benches wait at numerous locations.

TRAIL DESCRIPTION:

Begin at the **Harris Dr.** trailhead at the southern end where the trail extends northward along the grassy shoulder of **Winsted Rd.** After a half-mile, it separates from the road with a buffer of trees and, just ahead, gets its first view of the **Still River** on the right at the crossing of **South Rd.**

The trail continues along the river bank and intersects **North Rd.**, crosses a bridge over a tributary stream, and reaches the village of **Burrville** at **Greenwoods Rd.** (1.1 miles). After crossing, it follows the entrance to a trailhead parking lot for a short distance before resuming. A portable toilet is located at this trailhead in the warm season.

The next half-mile parallels the river and its open wetland. The trail comes alongside Winsted Rd. and

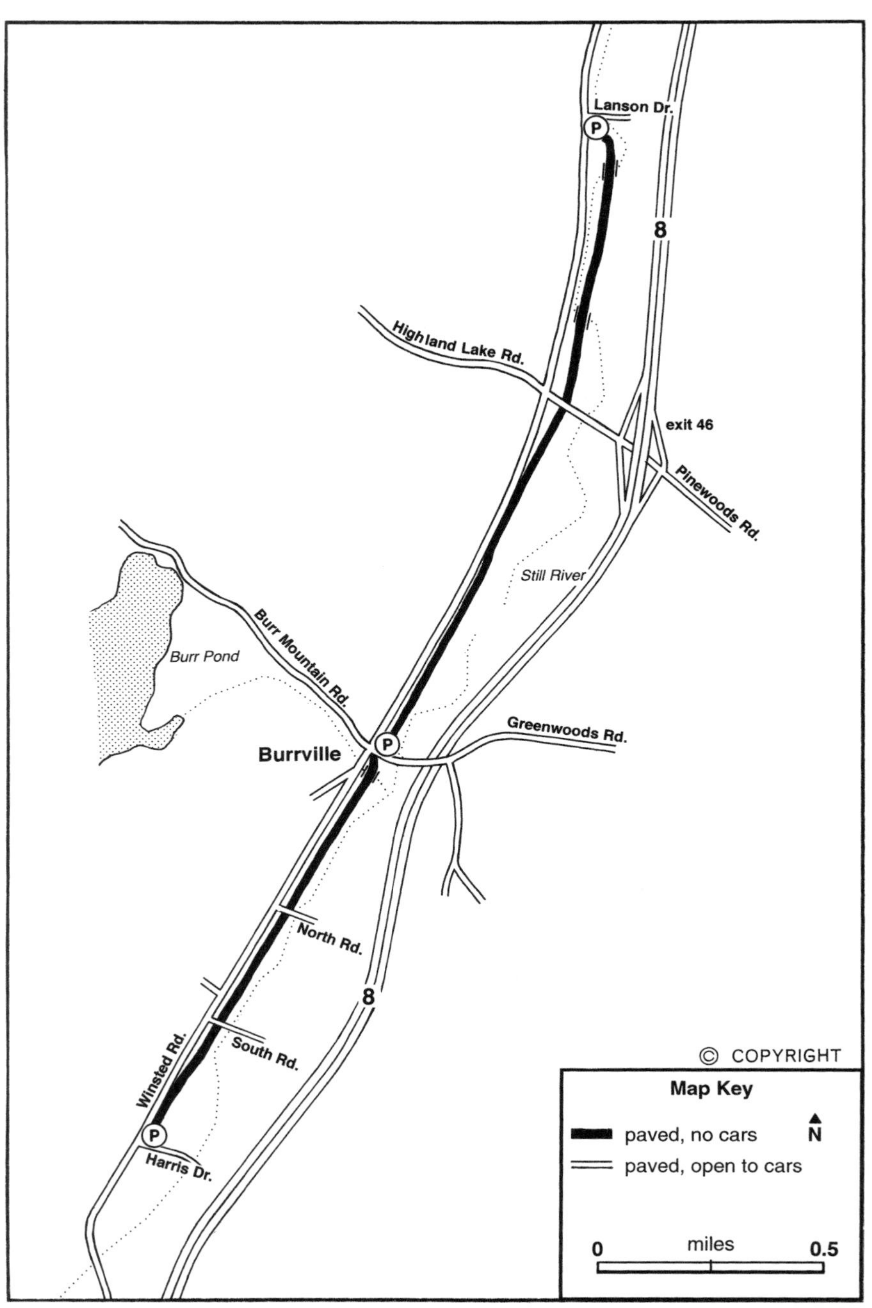
Lanson Dr.
P
8
Highland Lake Rd.
exit 46
Pinewoods Rd.
Still River
Burr Pond
Burr Mountain Rd.
Burrville
P
Greenwoods Rd.
North Rd.
8
South Rd.
Winsted Rd.
P
Harris Dr.
© COPYRIGHT
Map Key
paved, no cars
paved, open to cars
N
0
miles
0.5

crosses the driveways for several businesses along the way, then veers from the roadside and enjoys a few more glimpses of the river through leafy surroundings.

It intersects **Pinewoods Rd.** at the 2.1-mile mark near a memorial for Sue Grossman, an important advocate for the creation of the greenway, and a sign recognizing other trail supporters. Continuing, it crosses a bridge over the Still River (2.3 miles), straightens along the opposite bank where it meets the Winchester town line, and then crosses another bridge over the river. Just ahead, the trail ends at a trailhead parking area off **Lanson Dr.** (2.8 miles) in Winchester.

BACKGROUND:

The greenway follows the route of the Naugatuck Railroad which was completed in 1849 between Devon and Winsted. The railroad thrived on the transportation needs of local industries but its prosperity eventually declined with the 1900's. Passenger service along this stretch of the line ended in 1958 and the railroad was abandoned in 1963.

The rail bed lay dormant for decades until its rebirth as a recreational trail. Following years of effort, the greenway opened in 2009 and is dedicated to Sue Grossman, an important benefactor and advocate for its creation. Future construction is expected to extend the trail northward for two miles in Winchester and southward to Kennedy Dr. in Torrington.

DRIVING DIRECTIONS:

Harris Dr. trailhead from Rte. 8 northbound: Take Exit 45, turn left (west) on Kennedy Dr., then right (north) on Winsted Rd. Drive for 1.6 miles, turn right on Harris Dr., then immediately left at the trailhead parking lot.

Harris Dr. trailhead from Rte. 8 southbound: Take Exit 45, turn right (north) on Winsted Rd. After 1.9 miles, turn right on Harris Dr. then left at the trailhead parking lot.

Lanson Dr. trailhead from Rte. 8: Take Exit 46 and follow Pinewoods Rd. west for a quarter-mile, then turn right (north) on Winsted Rd. and continue for 0.6 miles. Turn right on Lanson Dr., then immediately right at the parking area.

TOILETS:

portable toilet at Greenwoods Rd. in Burrville (in season)

ADDITIONAL INFORMATION:

www.torringtontrails.webs.com

10 Edgewood Park

New Haven

LENGTH: 1.2 miles
SURFACE: paved
TERRAIN: mostly flat with one hill

This short, scenic stretch of car-free pavement provides welcome greenspace for the surrounding city.

RULES & SAFETY:

- The park is heavily used so bicyclists should ride with caution and be courteous to others.
- Ride at a safe speed and use extra caution in the presence of children and pets.
- Bicycling is permitted only on paved surfaces and is prohibited on unpaved trails.
- Help keep it clean: carry out all that you carry in.
- Dogs must be leashed and their wastes removed.
- The park is open from sunrise to sunset.

ORIENTATION:

Surrounded by residential streets, Edgewood Park stands as an oasis of greenspace along the West River. The park's only paved route runs from the parking lot and tennis courts in the north to the ranger station in the south.

TRAIL DESCRIPTION:

Starting at the parking lot off **West Rock Ave.**, follow the paved pathway leading into woods from the left side of the tennis courts. It crosses the **West River** on a low, arched bridge and soon ends at the park's main road.

Turn right and follow its broad surface south past the **Coogan Pavilion** where a half-pipe and array of ramps entertrain skateboarders. The road follows a strip of shaded lawns, enters a wooded area along the river, and passes under **Edgewood Ave.** at a multi-arched bridge. It bends left at a broad lawn surrounding **Duck Pond** and then begins to climb a noticeable slope, curving through a tree-covered

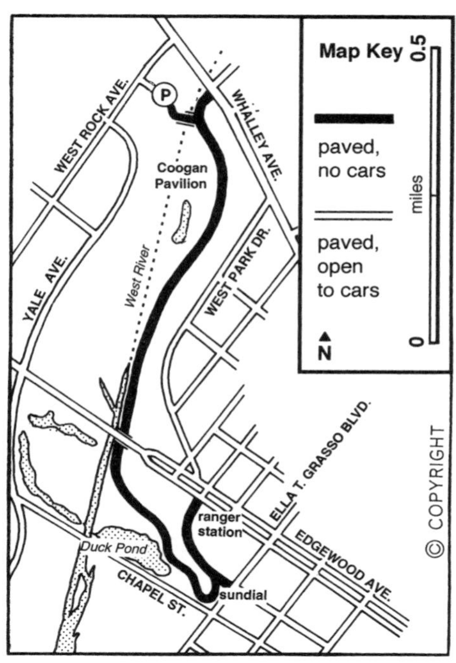

area to the edge of **Chapel St.** where it reverses direction with a long curve back to the north.

Just ahead, the road reaches a T-intersection at the **sundial** near a park entrance at **Ella T. Grasso Blvd.** Turn left at this intersection to ride the last stretch of pavement, a crescent-shaped road which returns to Edgewood Ave. near the **ranger station**.

BACKGROUND:

The donation of this land in 1889 created one of the city's first public parks and inspired the acquisition of other properties by the city's newly formed Park Commission. It was developed with input from Frederick Law Olmsted in 1910 and Beatrix Farrand in 1937.

DRIVING DIRECTIONS:

From I-95 take Exit 47 (or if southbound on I-91 take Exit 1) and follow Rte. 34 west for 1.9 miles, then continue on Rte. 10 north for 1.6 miles. Where Rte. 10 turns right on Fitch Ave., continue straight on Rte. 63 (Whalley Ave.) for a tenth of a mile, turn left on West Rock Ave., and find the parking lot just ahead on the left.

From Rte. 15 (Merritt Pkwy.), take Exit 59 and follow Rte. 69 south for a quarter-mile. Merge with Rte. 63 south and continue for 1.3 miles, then turn right on West Rock Ave. The parking lot is just ahead on the left.

TOILETS:

ranger station, Coogan Pavilion

ADDITIONAL INFORMATION:

New Haven Dept. of Parks, Rec., & Trees, (203) 946-8021

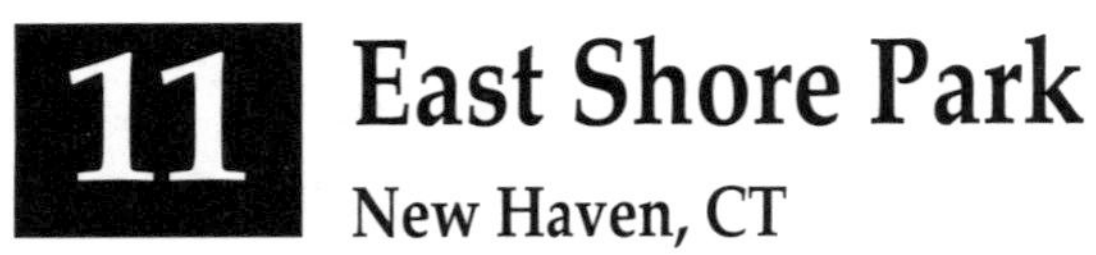

11 East Shore Park

New Haven, CT

LENGTH: 2 miles
SURFACE: paved
TERRAIN: flat

A steady breeze off the harbor helps keep this small cluster of pathways cool in summer.

RULES & SAFETY:

- Bicyclists should yield to pedestrians.
- Alert others (*"On your left..."*) when approaching from behind to avoid startling them.
- Move off the trail when stopped so others can pass.
- Help keep it clean: carry out all that you carry in.
- Dogs must be leashed and their wastes removed.
- The park is open from sunrise to sunset.

ORIENTATION:

The park's paved trail network has many intersections but its small scale and open landscape make it easy to find your way. The trails are bound by athletic facilities to the east and by the harbor to the west.

TRAIL DESCRIPTION:

Several trails explore the area between the baseball fields and tennis courts but the most popular and scenic path is the mile-long loop starting near the main parking lot.

Following it in the clockwise direction, ride past the trailhead gate heading west from the parking lot (toward the harbor) and keep straight on the trail that soon curves left (south) beside an access road and the baseball fields.

At 0.2 miles, continue straight (south) at a four-way intersection where the trail enters a broader area of lawns. After another 0.2 miles, the trail turns back toward the harbor and then follows the shoreline northward. The path enters a circle of pavement where a ring of benches are stationed, then snakes through trees as it progresses northward. A

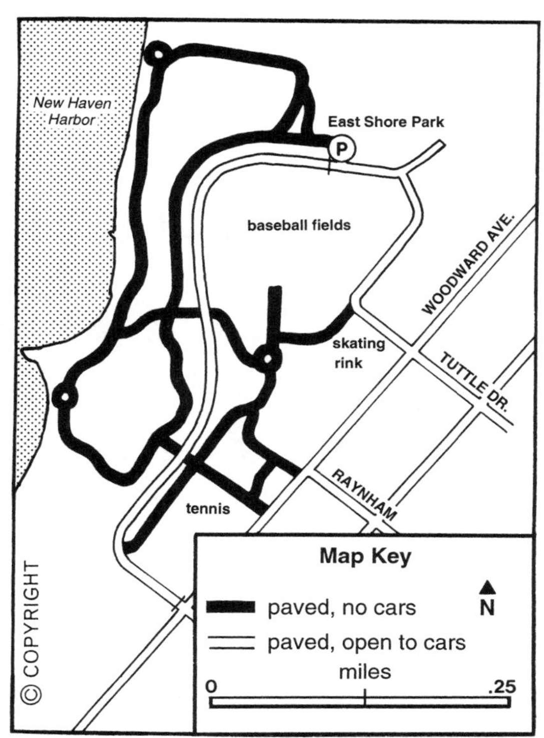

natural hedge of bushes blocks many of the water views at first but the trail eventually gains full exposure to the harbor and its breezes.

It reaches a second ring of benches at the 0.8-mile mark and turns inland. Heading east, the trail slips between a soccer field and the park's northern boundary fence and returns to the start of the loop at the trailhead gate and parking lot.

BACKGROUND:

This land was deeded to the city in 1923. When New Haven Harbor was dredged in 1941, much of the excavated material was dumped at East Shore Park to fill its wetlands and create usable recreation space. Additional work in the 1970's and 1980's established the park's lawns and tree plantings as well as an array of recreational facilities which includes the paved bike paths.

DRIVING DIRECTIONS:

• **From I-95 northbound:** Take Exit 50 and drive south on Woodward Ave. for 0.8 miles. Turn right at the park's entrance and continue to the parking lot at the end of the drive.

• **From I-95 southbound:** Take Exit 51 and follow Rte. 1 west for 0.9 miles. Turn left on Woodward Ave. and drive for 0.8 miles, then turn right at the park's entrance. Continue to the parking lot at the end of the drive.

TOILETS:

beside the ice skating rink

ADDITIONAL INFORMATION:

New Haven Parks, Rec., & Trees, (203) 946-8021

12 East Rock Park

New Haven - Hamden, CT

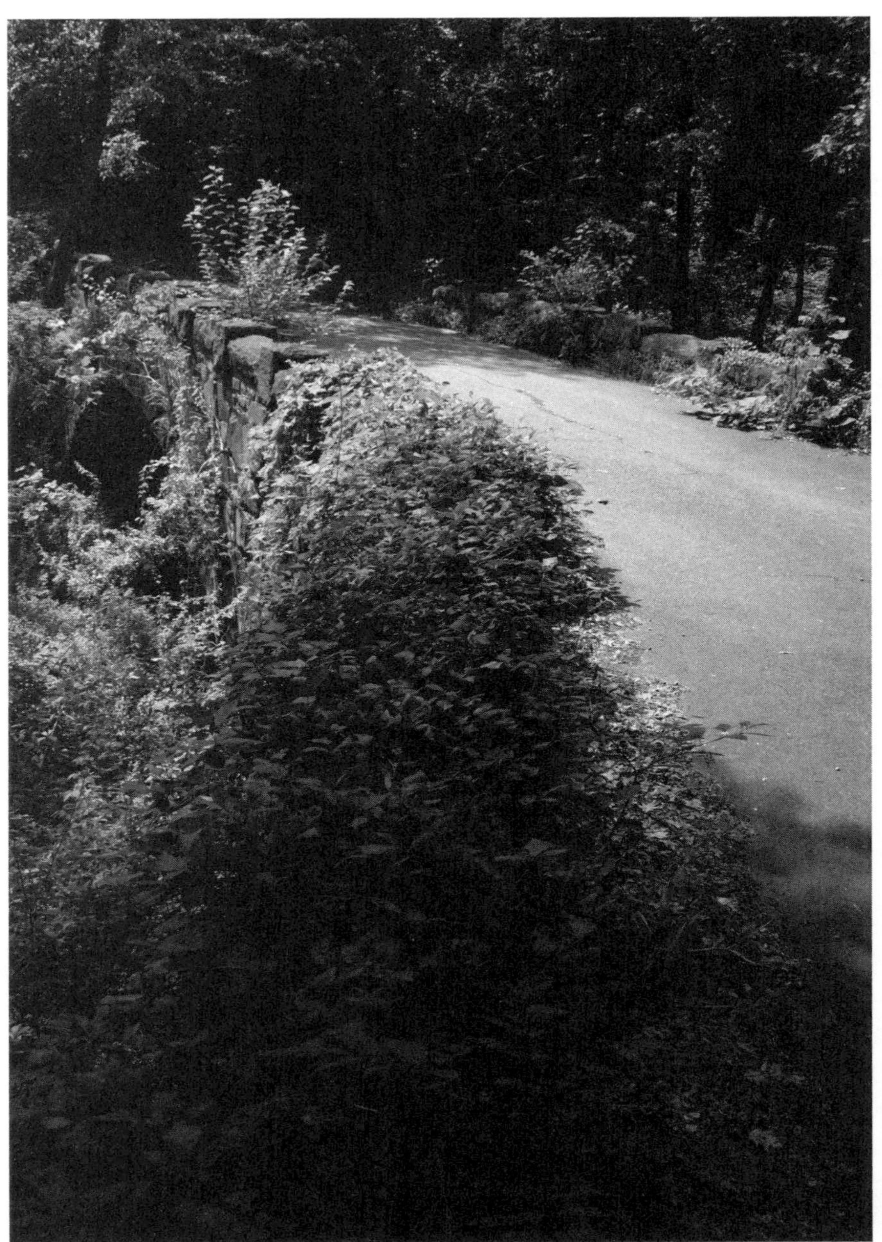

LENGTH: 2.3 miles
SURFACE: paved
TERRAIN: hilly
NOTE: not suitable for in-line skating

East Rock Park's carriage roads curve gracefully over stone arch bridges and climb to a bird's eye view over New Haven. Mountainous terrain makes them challenging to ride.

RULES & SAFETY:

- Bicycles are permitted only on the paved roads, and are prohibited from the unpaved trails.
- Two of the park's roads are sometimes open to cars. Hillhouse Dr. and the upper end of Farnam Dr. are open to car traffic for most of the year, but are closed to cars Monday-Thursday (excluding holidays) from November 1 to March 31.
- The roads are steep and curvy. Ride at a safe speed, keep to the right side, and be ready to encounter others.
- Alert others (*"On your left..."*) when approaching from behind to avoid startling them.
- Help keep it clean: carry out all that you carry in.
- Dogs must be leashed and their wastes removed.
- The park is open from sunrise to sunset.

ORIENTATION:

East Rock Park has dramatic topography. The roads turn frequently in order to negotiate this terrain and they can easily disorient newcomers, while their steepness will test the physical limits of some bicyclists.

The straightest, mildest option is Trowbridge Dr. while hillier, curvier conditions await on English, Farnam, and Hilhouse drives. Although parallel segments of these roads appear on the map to lie close together, very steep terrain separates them.

Road names are not posted so visitors are encouraged to bring a map when exploring the park for the first time. Trailhead parking is recommended at North Meadow on Farnam Dr. at the north end of the park.

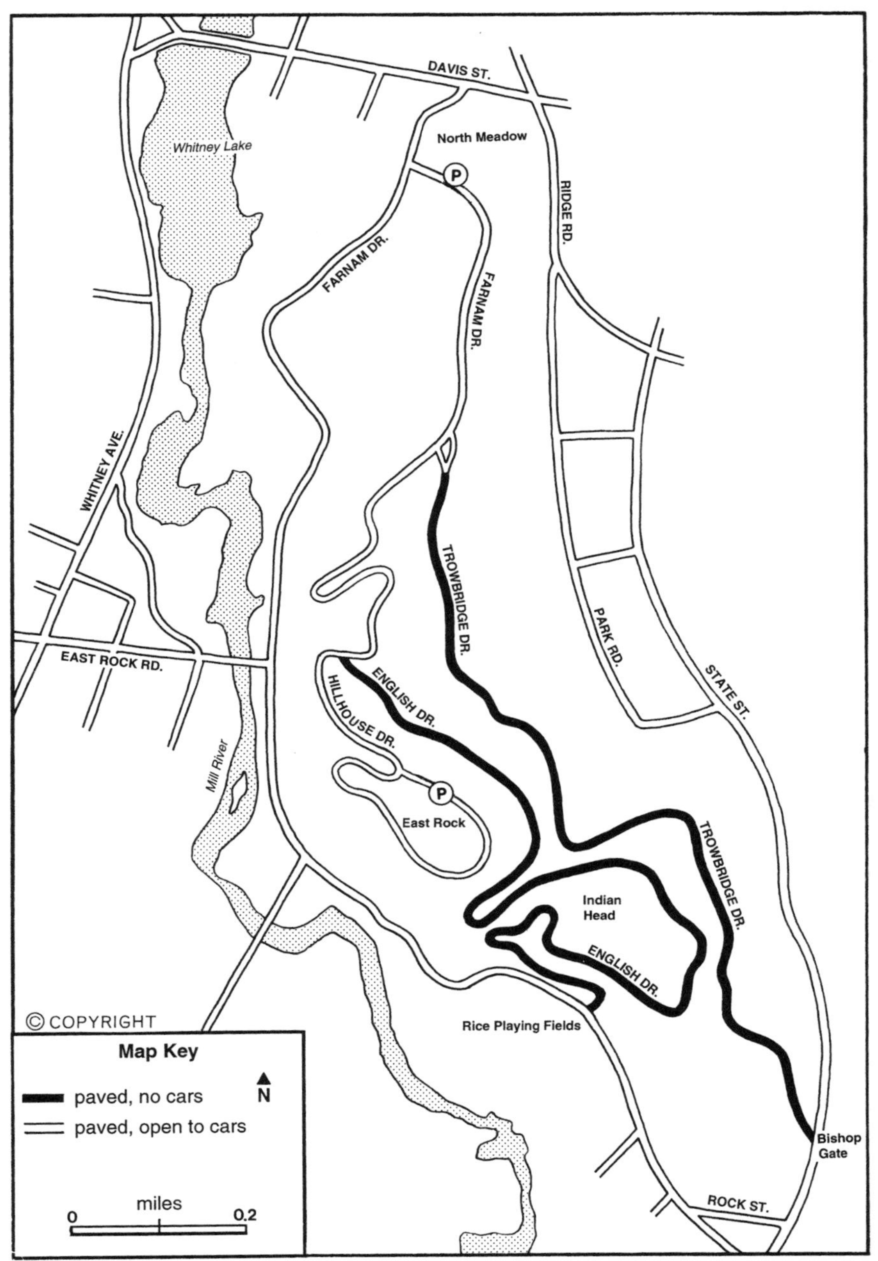
DAVIS ST.
North Meadow
Whitney Lake
RIDGE RD.
FARNAM DR.
FARNAM DR.
WHITNEY AVE.
TROWBRIDGE DR.
PARK RD.
EAST ROCK RD.
ENGLISH DR.
HILLHOUSE DR.
STATE ST.
Mill River
East Rock
TROWBRIDGE DR.
Indian Head
ENGLISH DR.
Rice Playing Fields
Bishop Gate
ROCK ST.
© COPYRIGHT
Map Key
paved, no cars
paved, open to cars
N
miles
0
0.2

TRAIL DESCRIPTION:

Farnam Dr. continues uphill from the trailhead parking lot at the northern end of the park and leads toward the summit. The road is closed to car traffic from November 1 to March 31 on Mondays, Tuesdays, Wednesdays, and Thursdays (excluding holidays), and attracts light traffic during the remaining periods when it is open to cars. The speed limit is posted at 25 m.p.h.

Farnam Dr. leaves the open air of **North Meadow** and enters the shade of woods where mature rhododendron bushes adorn the roadside and various groundcover plants carpet the forest floor. After a third of a mile of gentle incline, Farnam Dr. forks right at the intersection of Trowbridge Dr. and then gets steeper, curving through a switchback turn with an open view.

It ends at the 0.8-mile mark at the intersection of English Dr. Here **Hillhouse Dr.** continues the uphill tack for the remaining quarter-mile to the summit of **East Rock** (elevation 365') where cyclists can catch their breath while gazing over the sight of New Haven and its harbor. A broad lawn, parking lot, and war memorial occupy this high point.

Mile-long **Trowbridge Dr.** begins from Farnam Dr. a third of a mile up from the parking lot at North Meadow and takes a gradual downhill route to **State St.** at the southeast corner of the park. Closed to car traffic year-round, it is perhaps the least used of the park's paved roads so accummulated leaves and twigs give its surface a forgotten look.

Trowbridge starts with a taste of grandeur by crossing a stone arch bridge over a stream gulley, then continues along a flat course while turning frequently with the side of a slope. Here the road's flat profile and smooth surface stand in marked contrast to the surrounding terrain which appears rocky and mountainous. More rhododendrons and mountain laurel bushes, planted during the park's early days, grow beside the road with sprawling, contorted limbs. A slight downhill grade develops after a half-mile and, after a right-hand corner, the road comes within sight and sound of State St. The remaining distance to **Bishop Gate** has a moderate downslope and meandering curves.

English Dr. has steeper hills and sharper turns. Beginning at the intersection of Farnam and Hillhouse drives near the summit of East Rock, it descends for 1.3 miles to the base elevation at **Rock St.** After the first 0.4 miles of gradual descent, the road emerges from the forest shade at the bottom of an open cliff face below the summit, reverses direction at a hair-pin turn, and begins to circle the smaller hilltop known as **Indian Head**.

English Dr. comes within sight of Trowbridge Dr. at a few points along this distance but a steep slope forms a barrier between the two routes. Halfway around Indian Head the road crosses a large stone arch bridge and then begins a final, half-mile descent which holds steeper pitches and several switchback corners. Limited visibility warrants slow speeds for cyclists along this portion of the road. Car-free pavement ends at a gate at the bottom of the hill on Rock St. across from the **Rice Playing Fields**.

BACKGROUND:

Proposals to establish East Rock as a public park date from 1877 when Noah Porter, president of Yale College, sparked the creation of a commission to acquire and manage the land. Over the next fifty years, the commission was able to succeed in this effort with the help of donations of both land and money.

The park now totals 425 acres and has a variety of features. Four carriage roads were created with donated funds in the park's early days and are now a highlight for visitors who can reach the summit by car or explore other areas that are closed to traffic. A 112' monument at the top, visible from miles away, was built in 1887 to honor soldiers who died in the Revolutionary War, the War of 1812, the Mexican War, and the Civil War. Athletic fields, 10 miles of hiking trails, picnic areas, and playgrounds are among the other attractions.

DRIVING DIRECTIONS:

From I-91 take Exit 6. Turn left off the ramp on Willow St., then immediately left on State St. and continue for 1.4 miles to a traffic signal at Ridge Rd. Turn left on Ridge Rd. and continue for 0.4 miles, bear left on Davis St., then left at the park entrance. Take the first left to reach the parking lot on Farnam Dr.

From Rte. 15 (Merritt Pkwy.) take Exit 61 and turn south on Whitney Ave. following signs to New Haven. Continue on Whitney Ave. for 2.8 miles and then turn left on Davis St. and drive for a half-mile. Turn right at the park entrance, then take the first left to reach the Farnam Dr. parking lot.

TOILETS:

the ranger station on Orange St., in season

ADDITIONAL INFORMATION:

New Haven Dept. of Parks, Rec., & Trees, (203) 946-8021
East Rock Ranger Station, (203) 946-6086
Park Security Office, (203) 946-7268

13 West Rock Ridge State Park

New Haven - Hamden, CT

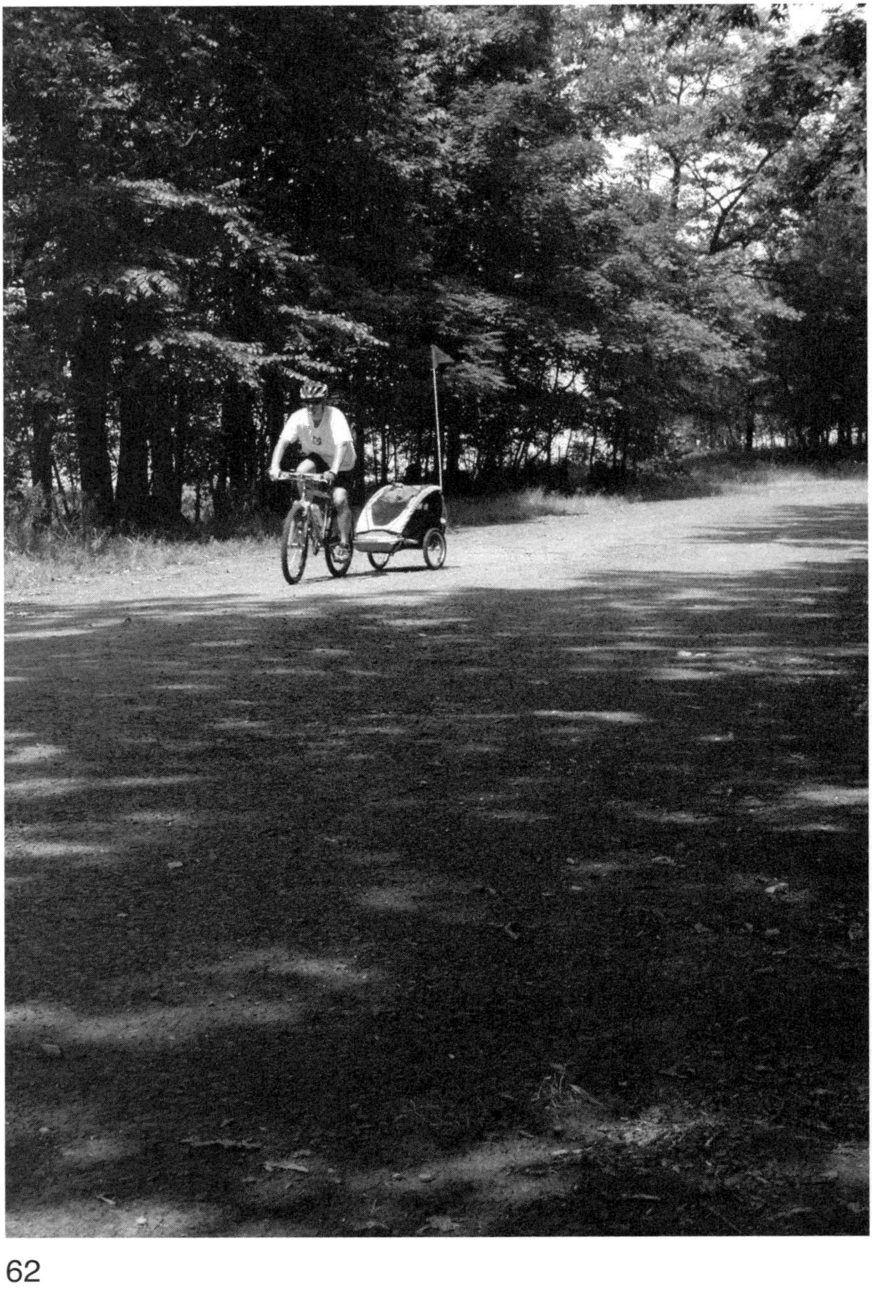

LENGTH: 8.5 miles
SURFACE: mostly paved
TERRAIN: hilly
NOTE: not suitable for in-line skating

After a sizeable uphill climb, this gated park road delivers a quiet, ridgeline ride with natural surroundings and distant views. Nearby, an unpaved loop circles a small lake with gentler slopes.

RULES & SAFETY:

- Bicyclists should yield to pedestrians.
- Ride at a safe speed, keep to the right side, and alert others (*"On your left..."*) when approaching from behind.
- Use extra caution on the steep, hairpin corners of Baldwin Dr., and remember that other cyclists, walkers, and work vehicles could appear at any moment.
- Note that access to Baldwin Dr. is limited to the two end points.
- Help keep it clean: carry out all that you carry in.
- Dogs must be leashed and their wastes removed.
- The park is open from 8:00AM until sunset.
- Watch for additional regulations posted at trailheads.

ORIENTATION:

Aside from the park's mountain biking trails, three options exist for bicyclists. The seldom-used northern leg of Baldwin Dr. offers a 5.6-mile, car-free roadway that ascends a steep slope and then follows the flat, forested crest of West Rock Ridge with viewpoints at intervals along the way. The southern leg of Baldwin Dr. is open to cars during the warm season and climbs for 1.2 miles to a panoramic view of New Haven at South Overlook. Both of these roads are accessed from the Nature Center parking lot across Wintergreen Ave.

A third option circles Lake Wintergreen from a trailhead on Main St. with milder terrain in the park's lower elevations. An unpaved, 1.6-mile loop, this improved trail gets regular usage from walkers and runners and offers a smooth ride with several water views.

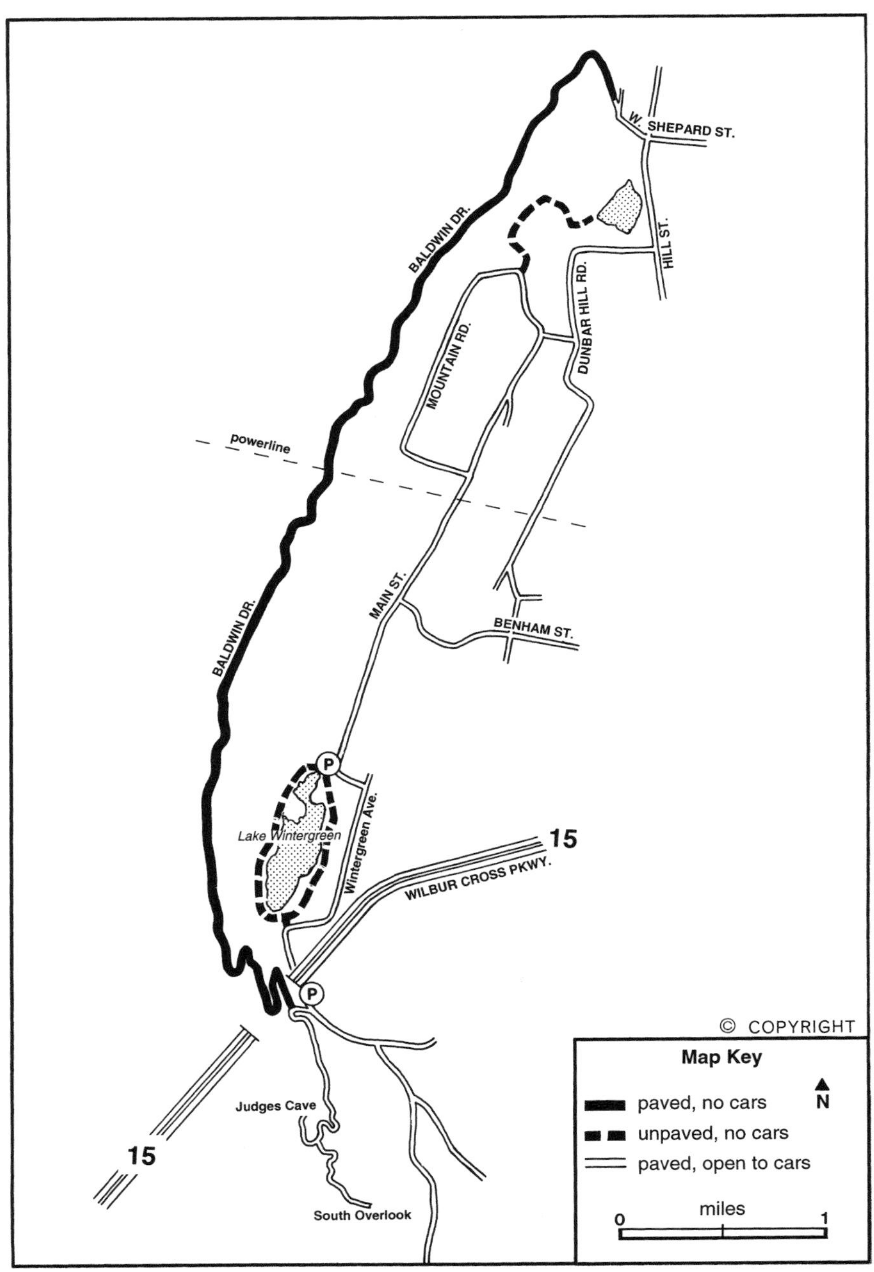
W. SHEPARD ST.
HILL ST.
BALDWIN DR.
DUNBAR HILL RD.
MOUNTAIN RD.
powerline
MAIN ST.
BENHAM ST.
BALDWIN DR.
P
Lake Wintergreen
Wintergreen Ave.
15
WILBUR CROSS PKWY.
P
© COPYRIGHT
Map Key
paved, no cars
unpaved, no cars
paved, open to cars
N
miles
0
1
Judges Cave
15
South Overlook

TRAIL DESCRIPTION:

Starting at the **Nature Center** parking lot, turn left on **Wintergreen Ave.** and look for the entrance to **Baldwin Dr.** on the right after a short distance. The road is named after Simeon Baldwin, governor of Connecticut from 1911 to 1915, who bequeathed funds for its construction in 1927.

Ride past the gate and turn right where the road forks at the base of the hill. Heading north, this 5.6-mile stretch of roadway climbs immediately with a strenuous, 0.8-mile incline which provides brief respites at a few hairpin corners. The paved surface, cracking with age and narrowing from encroaching foliage, has an abandoned look but bicyclists should stay alert for other riders, walkers, and the possibility of a work vehicle sharing the road. The initial pitch rises past the entrance to the **Wilbur Cross Pkwy.** tunnel and the first switchback corner, reached in less than a quarter-mile. After much effort, the road gains the top of the ridge a short distance beyond the third switchback and offers a western view before turning a final time to the north.

Baldwin Dr. straightens at this point on a relatively flat, 0.6-mile segment which is shaded by hardwood forest. (Note that a few footpaths diverge on the left (west) side of the road to reach the top of an open cliff face where extreme caution should be used.) A downward slope follows this straightaway and allows cyclists to coast for a quarter-mile before the road tilts uphill on an incline which lasts for about a half-mile.

Another mile of relatively flat and straight riding ensues before the road rises on a short uphill, crosses a set of **powerlines**, and begins a rolling, up-and-down course for the remaining 2.5 miles. Turnouts in the pavement mark several viewpoints along the way. At the end, the road drops on one of its steepest slopes, turns to the south at a barricade blocking vehicle entry, and descends to the end of **West Shepard St.**

The southern leg of Baldwin Dr. is shorter, more heavily visited, and open to cars during the warm season.

Forking left at the bottom near the entrance gate, the road climbs at an easier pace for 0.7 miles to a second fork. Turning left again, riders ascend for another half-mile to **South Overlook** where an unobstructed view spreads southward over New Haven and Long Island Sound. Turning right, riders soon reach **Judges Cave**, a formation of boulders where in 1661 two members of Parliament hid from officers of the Crown after signing a death warrant of King Charles I.

The popular loop around **Lake Wintergreen** is not flat but the hills are much smaller than those on Baldwin Dr. The unpaved trail is 1.6 miles long, has a smooth surface which varies between crushed stone and packed dirt, and offers views of the lake at numerous points.

Following it in the clockwise direction from the parking lot on **Main St.**, face downhill and turn immediately left on the trail that extends southward in a straight line for a quarter-mile. It rises over a knoll, forks left at a dam containing the lake, and descends below the dam and into woods. After passing a service building beside **Wintergreen Ave.** at the south end of the lake, the trail scrambles up its steepest hill and proceeds straight through a four-way intersection on its return to the north. The last leg measures three quarters of a mile and features gently rolling terrain with glimpses of the lake through the trees. Turn right at the next four-way intersection, cross a bridge over Wintergreen Brook, and climb the slope to return to the trailhead parking lot.

BACKGROUND:

The first settlers found the terrain around West Rock Ridge to be too rough for farming but made good use of its timber, firewood, and stone. As the surrounding population grew and open space dwindled, West Rock became a popular place for residents to enjoy the outdoors and by the late 1800's visitors were ascending a new carriage road to the top of the hill and marveling at the distant views.

The state formed this 1500-acre park in 1977 by uniting parcels of land previously owned by the city of New Haven, the South Central Regional Water Authority, and others.

DRIVING DIRECTIONS:

Lake Wintergreen trailhead: From Rte. 15 (Wilbur Cross Pkwy.) take Exit 60 and follow Rte. 10 south, then turn right on Benham St. and drive for 2 miles to the end. Turn left on Main St. and look for the Lake Wintergreen trailhead parking lot 0.5 miles ahead on the right at a sharp, left-hand turn.

Baldwin Dr. trailhead: As above, then continue on Main St. for a short distance to the end. Turn right on Wintergreen Ave. and look for the Nature Center parking lot on the left after the road passes underneath the Wilbur Cross Pkwy. The entrance to Baldwin Dr. is a short distance ahead on the right.

TOILETS:

Lake Wintergreen trailhead

ADDITIONAL INFORMATION:

West Rock Ridge State Park, c/o Sleeping Giant State Park, (203) 789-7498

14 Quinnipiac River Linear Trail

Wallingford

LENGTH: 1.2 miles
SURFACE: paved
TERRAIN: flat

Wallingford's short bike path is flat and free of any road intersections so it's ideal for young kids. Noise from a nearby highway detracts from otherwise natural scenery.

RULES & SAFETY:

• Bicyclists should yield to pedestrians.

• Keep to the right, pass on the left, and alert others (*"On your left..."*) when approaching from behind.

• Dogs must be leashed and their wastes removed.

• The trail is open from dawn to dusk.

ORIENTATION:

The dead end trail has only one point of entry and requires an out-and-back ride. It is confined by parallel Rte. 15 (Wilbur Cross Pkwy.) on one side and the Quinnipiac River on the other and, with the exception of the highway, encounters no signs of civilization.

TRAIL DESCRIPTION:

The trail begins at **Hall Ave.** (**Rte. 150**), circles the recreation area and trailhead near **Community Lake** for the first 0.2 miles, then enters woods paralleling the **Wilbur Cross Pkwy.** (**Rte. 15**) for the remaining mile.

Dense brush blocks most views until the midpoint. After crossing a stream, the trail passes the **Emerson J. Leonard Wildlife Sanctuary**, a 20-acre tract which preserves natural scenery on the right. A third of a mile ahead, a plaque on the left honors one of the state's largest oak trees which stands nearby.

Near the end, the trail reaches a turnout at a small clearing beside the **Quinnipiac River** where several benches invite a rest, then continues across the water on a

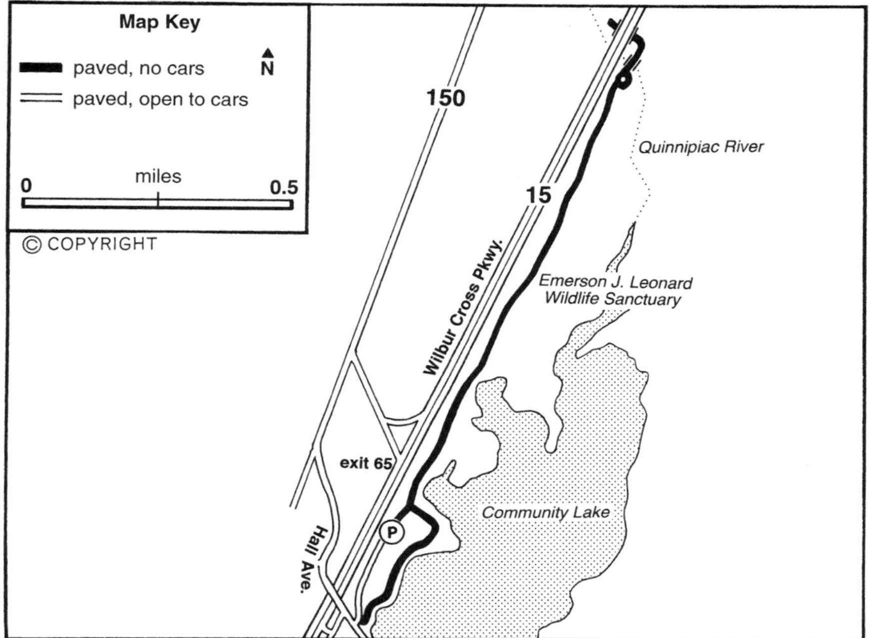

bike/pedestrian bridge. On the other side, it continues through a tunnel under Rte. 15 and then ends abruptly.

BACKGROUND:

Opened in 2000, the trail is a creation of the Quinnipiac River Linear Trail Advisory Committee which was established in 1997 to create a linear park along the river for not only trail users but also canoeists and others. Future construction is proposed along a 7-mile route through Wallingford between Meriden and North Haven.

DRIVING DIRECTIONS:

From the Wilbur Cross Pkwy. (Rte. 15), take Exit 65. If southbound, turn left off the ramp and follow Rte. 150 south for a half-mile, cross over the highway, and turn left at the park entrance. If northbound, keep left at the end of the ramp and continue straight across Rte. 150 to enter the park.

TOILETS:

portable at Community Lake trailhead

ADDITIONAL INFORMATION:

Quinnipiac River Linear Trail Advisory Committee, Wallingford Town Hall, 45 S. Main St., Wallingford, CT 06492

15 Quinnipiac River Gorge Tr.

Meriden, CT

LENGTH: 1.3 miles
SURFACE: paved
TERRAIN: flat

Explore the Gorge Trail on a hot summer day and you'll love its cool shade and soothing river views. Since it crosses no roads, it's an ideal choice for a ride with children.

RULES & SAFETY:

- Bicyclists should yield to pedestrians.
- Keep to the right, pass on the left, and alert others (*"On your left..."*) when approaching from behind.
- Use extra caution when children or pets are present.
- Pets must be leashed and their wastes removed.
- The trail is open dawn-dusk, but can be closed during inclement weather.
- Signs warn of a falling-rock zone along one section.
- Parents of children should note that the railings of the Red Bridge (eastern endpoint) provide minimal protection.

ORIENTATION:

The trail has an east-west alignment with trailheads at both ends. Note that it intersects no other roads and is confined by the Quinnipiac River on one side and steep slopes on the other. The eastern trailhead, with additional parking across Oregon Rd., is the recommended starting point.

Future trail construction is expected to extend across Oregon Rd. and northward beside Hanover Pond.

TRAIL DESCRIPTION:

Beginning at the **Oregon Rd.** trailhead near **Red Bridge**, the trail follows the **Quinnipiac River** upstream through woods. It passes the first of several historical displays before curving left into the gorge area where a

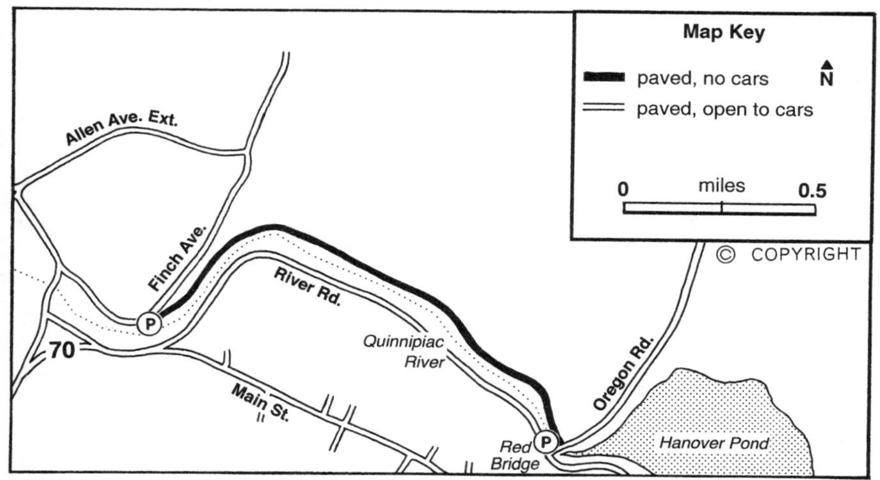

reddish siltstone cliff rises on the right side and the river flows rapidly over rocks on the left.

The cliffs recede at the 0.5-mile mark as the trail straightens for a while and then reappear and confine the trail to another narrow shelf along the riverbank. The trail passes the stone abuttments for the former High Bridge at the 1-mile mark, then exits the gorge and traverses flat woods for the last 0.3 miles to **Finch Ave.**

BACKGROUND:

This route originated in 1888 as the Meriden, Waterbury, and Connecticut River Railroad to serve the transportation needs of local industry. Service ended in 1917, the tracks were removed in 1929, and the route lay dormant until 2007 when it was reborn as a multi-use trail. Future construction is expected to extend the trail northward across Oregon Rd.

DRIVING DIRECTIONS:

From I-691 take Exit 4 and follow W. Main St. east for 2.2 miles. Turn south (right) on Oregon Rd. and drive for 1.5 miles to the end, turn right on River Rd., then immediately right at the parking lot. If it's full, reverse direction on Oregon Rd. and look for the larger lot on the right at Hanover Pond.

ADDITIONAL INFORMATION:

www.meridenlineartrail.org/Content/Quinnipiac_River_Gorge_Trail.asp

16 Farmington Canal Greenway

New Haven - Cheshire, CT

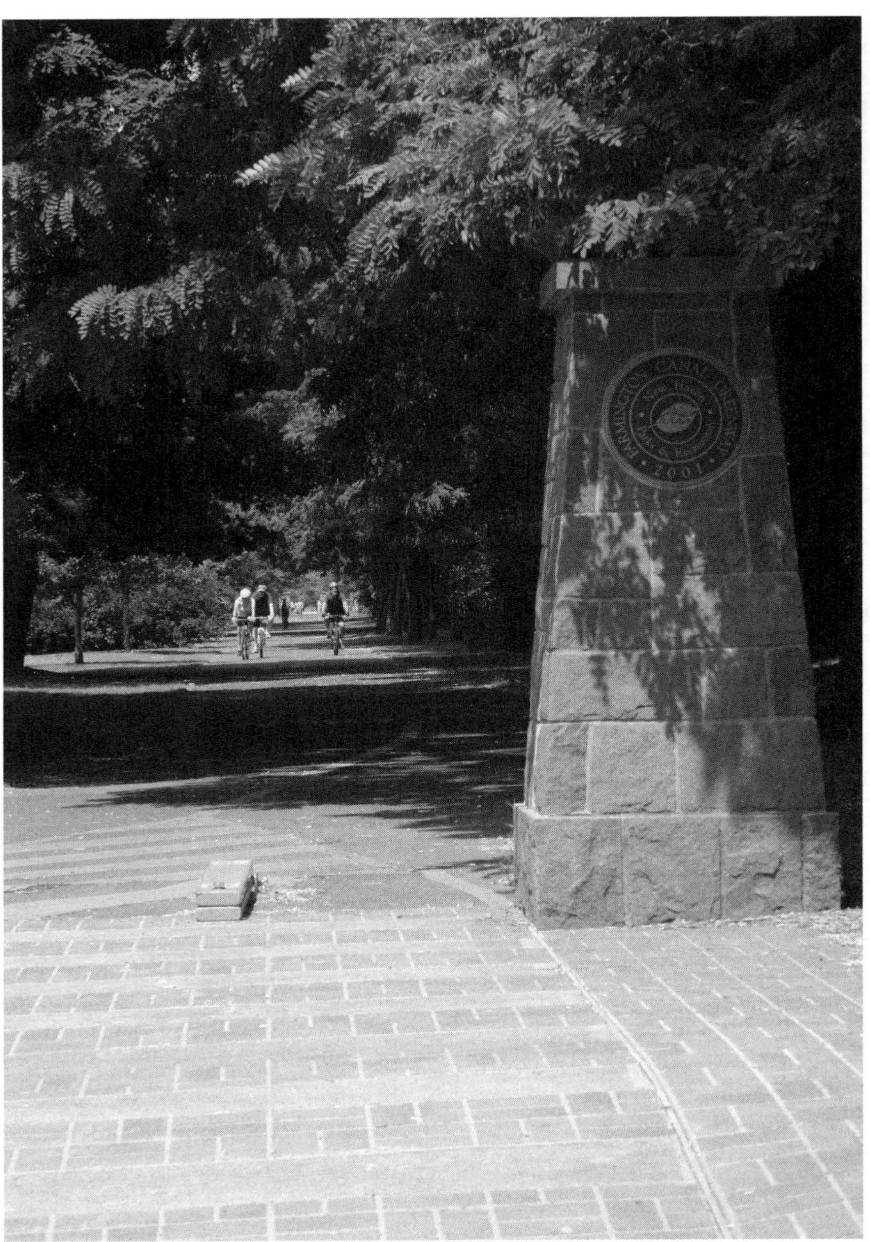

LENGTH: 14.4 miles
SURFACE: paved
TERRAIN: flat

One of Connecticut's most popular bike paths, this southern section of the historic Farmington Canal Greenway hosts a colorful parade of bicyclists, walkers, runners, and in-line skaters throughout the year.

RULES & SAFETY:

- Bicyclists should yield to pedestrians.
- Keep to the right, pass on the left, and alert others (*"On your left..."*) when approaching from behind.
- Ride at a safe speed. Be especially cautious in crowded areas, and in the presence of children and pets.
- Stop at road intersections and assume that drivers do not see you.
- Step off the trail when stopped to allow others to pass.
- Respect the private property along the trail.
- Help keep it clean: carry out all that you carry in.
- Dogs must be leashed and their wastes removed.
- The trail is open from dawn to dusk.

ORIENTATION:

This part of the greenway, known as the Farmington Canal Linear Park in Cheshire and the Farmington Canal Greenway in Hamden and New Haven, runs from Cornwall Ave. in Cheshire to Temple St. in New Haven. Other sections of the Farmington Greenway are described in chapters 17 and 18.

The trail's profile is generally flat with a slight pitch to the south. Exceptions to this are 3 detours from the original rail line in Hamden which encounter noticeable slopes.

Road intersections provide a useful means of plotting progress along the trail and are well equiped with stop signs, crosswalks, and metal posts to prevent vehicle entry. Trailheads are located in Cheshire and Hamden and include the popular Lock 12 Park near the trail's northern end where a picnic area, toilets, and drinking fountain are provided.

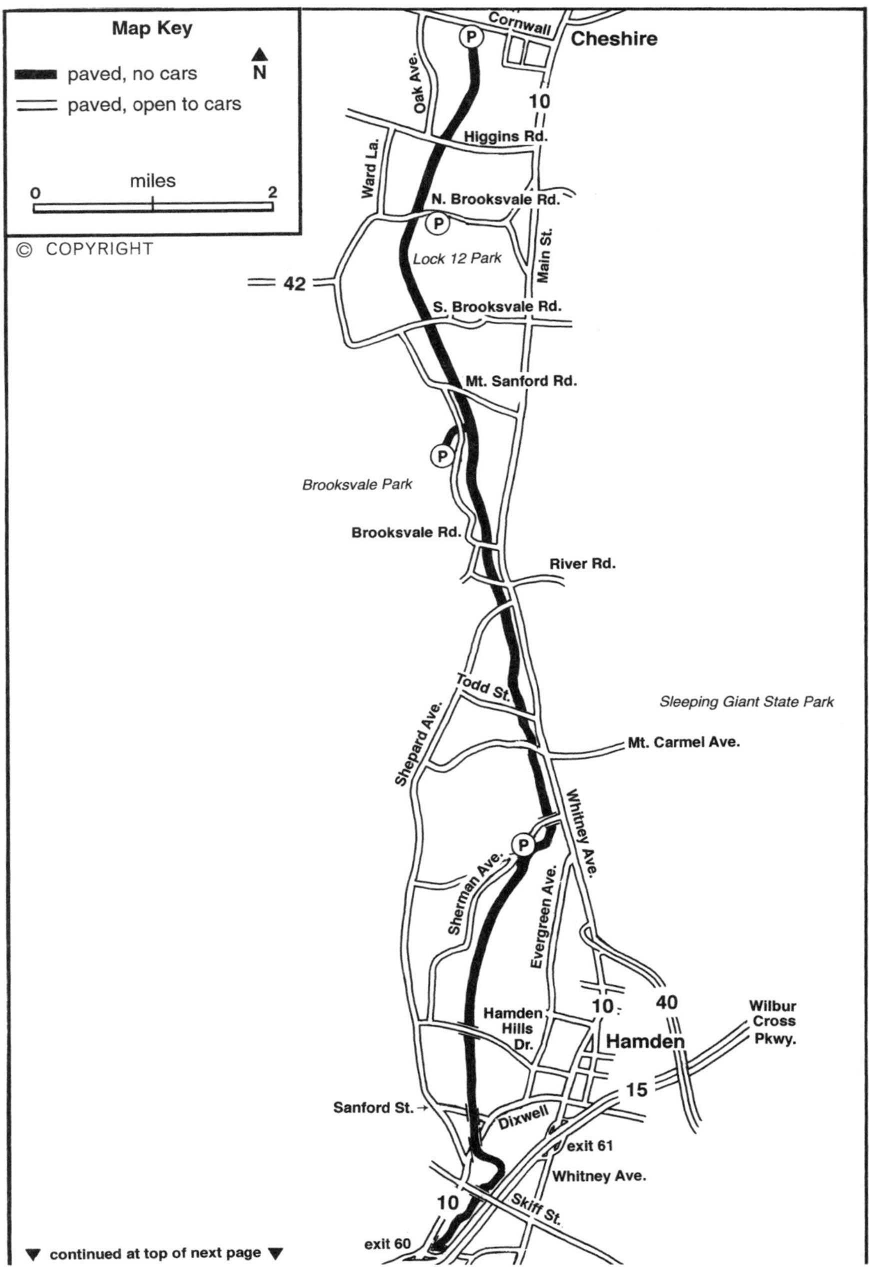

▼ continued at top of next page ▼

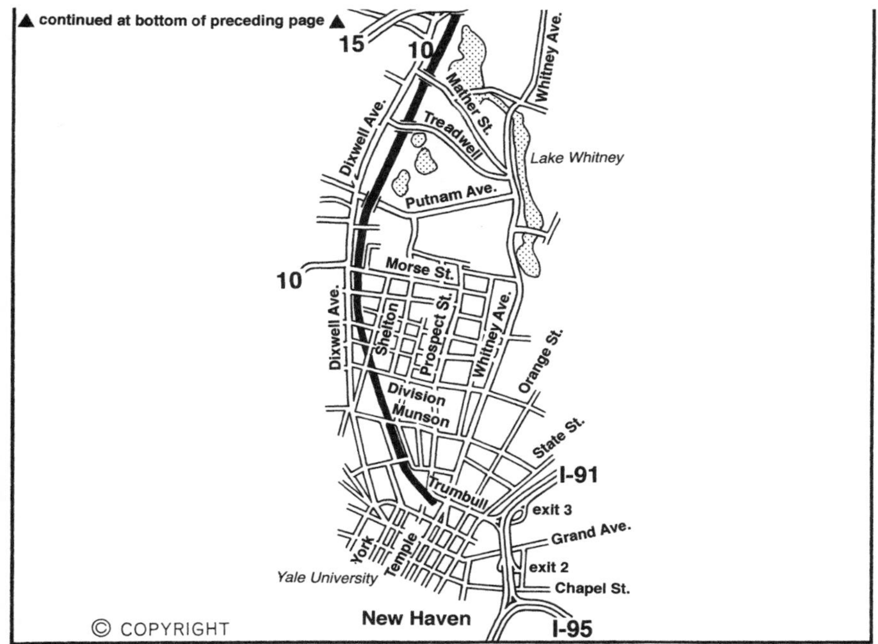

TRAIL DESCRIPTION:

Starting at **Lock 12 Park** on **North Brooksvale Rd.** (**Rte. 42**) in Cheshire, the trail extends in two directions. Heading north (from the parking lot, turning right), it runs for 1.6 miles along the canal bed with flat, shady conditions extending across **Higgins Rd.** to the end at **Cornwall Ave.** Heading south (from the parking lot, turning left), it extends for 12.8 miles beginning at a restored canal lock on the left side and a stone arch bridge over the canal.

The trail continues through woods along the water before emerging in a semi-open area at **South Brooksvale Rd.** (0.9 miles). It follows wooden fencing for the next half-mile to **Mt. Sanford Rd.** at the Hamden town line (1.4 miles) and passes a side trail on the right at the 1.7-mile mark leading to **Brooksvale Park**, a popular family destination offering a display of farm animals, a playground, hiking trails, and another option for trailhead parking.

The trail crosses **River Rd.** and **Shepard Ave.** within

the next half-mile, passes behind several businesses, and reaches a trailhead at **Todd St.** about 4.1 miles south of the Lock 12 Park trailhead. It then detours from the rail bed and drops to the side of busy **Whitney Ave.** (**Rte. 10**) where fencing and crosswalks guide the trail through a retail area and the intersection of **West Woods Rd.** (4.3 miles).

Rising on an uphill slope, the trail returns to the rail bed and begins a 6.4-mile leg which is free of intersections because bridges allow it to pass either over or under the roads encountered. (Note that side trails connect the greenway to many of these streets.) After passing under **Sherman Ave.** (5.0 miles) it makes a second detour, climbing past a trailhead and following the road for a quarter-mile before descending back to the rail bed.

The trail enjoys the shade of woods for the next few miles. It passes under **Hamden Hills Dr.** (6.7 miles) and follows the flow of a brook to a bridge over **Sanford St.** (7.3 miles). Just ahead, it passes over **Dixwell Ave.** (Rte. 10) (7.5 miles) and, at Hamden's commercial area, makes a final detour from the rail bed by descending a slope to the side of the **Merritt Pkwy.** and passing under **Skiff St.** (8.1 miles).

It skirts the back of a shopping area and returns to the rail bed, then crosses a bridge over **Connolly Pkwy.** (8.7 miles) and passes under the Merritt Pkwy. It straightens for the next 2 miles in back of a mixed retail and industrial area, enjoying the shade of woods bordering **Lake Whitney** as it passes under **Treadwell St.** (9.8 miles) and over **Putnam Ave.** (10.4 miles), the last of the bridged road intersections.

The trail enters a residential area at **Morse St.** (10.7 miles) where road intersections become more frequent. It intersects 10 roads in the next mile to **Division St.**, crossing the New Haven city line along the way. The scenery opens in another industrial area for the next half-mile and the trail gains a view of the New Haven skyline as it approaches **Munson St.** (12.2 miles). It continues beside Canal St. to the **Yale University** campus where the trail descends below grade and ends beneath **Temple St.** (12.8 miles).

BACKGROUND:

The Farmington Canal was completed between New Haven and Farmington in 1828 and extended to Northampton, MA in 1836 to facilitate commerce between the seaport and interior countryside. Over 80 miles in length, it was the longest canal ever built in New England and one of the most complex requiring 28 locks to meet changes in elevation, 13 culverts to allow streams to flow beneath the canal, 3 aqueducts to carry the canal over rivers, and 135 bridges for roads. The canal struggled to generate adequate revenues to repay these costs and closed in 1848 when a railroad began operation along the same route.

The railroad operated until 1982 when a flood destroyed a section of the line in Cheshire. A short time later, the Farmington Rail to Trail Association was established to convert the route to a bike path and by the mid-1990's the towns of Hamden and Cheshire had begun constructing the trail. It is a designated link of the East Coast Greenway, a 2600-mile multi-use trail from Maine to Florida.

DRIVING DIRECTIONS:

Lock 12 Park (Cheshire) from I-91: Take Exit 10 and follow Rte. 40 north for 2.5 miles to the end. Turn right on Rte. 10 north and continue for 5.9 miles, then turn left on Rte. 42 west. The park is 1 mile ahead on the left.

Lock 12 Park (Cheshire) from I-691: Take Exit 3 and follow Rte. 10 south to Cheshire. Turn right on Rte. 42 west and look for the park 1 mile ahead on the left.

Brooksvale Park (Hamden) from I-91: Take Exit 10 and follow Rte. 40 north for 2.5 miles to the end. Turn right on Rte. 10 north and continue for 3 miles, then turn left on Brooksvale Ave. The park is 0.7 miles ahead on the left.

Sherman Ave. (Hamden) from I-91: Take Exit 10 and follow Rte. 40 north for 2.5 miles to the end. Turn right on Rte. 10 north and continue for 0.9 miles, then turn left on Sherman Ave. Parking is at the top of the hill on the left.

Sherman Ave. (Hamden) from Wilbur Cross Pkwy. (Rte 15): Take Exit 60 and follow Rte. 10 north for 4.1 miles, turn left on Sherman Ave., and park ahead on the left.

TOILETS:

Lock 12 Park (Cheshire), Brooksvale Park (Hamden)

ADDITIONAL INFORMATION:

www.farmingtoncanal.org

17 Farmington Canal Greenway

Southington, CT

LENGTH: 3.9 miles
SURFACE: paved
TERRAIN: flat

Revival of this historic transportation route has created enjoyable greenspace and a smooth ribbon of asphalt through the heart of Southington's active industrial corridor.

RULES & SAFETY:

- Bicyclists and skaters should yield to pedestrians.
- Ride at a safe speed, especially when children or pets are present.
- Keep to the right, pass on the left, and alert others (*"On your left..."*) when approaching from behind.
- Step off the trail when stopped to allow others to pass.
- Help keep the trail clean and free of litter.
- Dogs must be leashed and under control, and their wastes removed.

ORIENTATION:

The trail is aligned in the north-south direction with two main trailhead parking lots located near each endpoint and additional parking spots located in between. Road intersections are numerous and some are busy with traffic, but crosswalks and signage are in place to safely guide trail travelers. Benches have been placed at several locations to allow visitors to stop and rest.

TRAIL DESCRIPTION:

Begin at the **Mill St.** trailhead parking lot near the northern end of the trail. Heading north (left), the trail enjoys green surroundings for its 0.6-mile distance to **Hart St.** where an old-fashioned sign reading *"New Haven & Northampton Railroad"* arches overhead as a reminder of the future long-distance possibilities for this greenway.

Farther north, the tracks remain in place beneath a cover of weeds and brush.

Heading south from Mill St., the trail runs for 3.3 miles with a view of Southington's industrial base and the crossing of two small rivers. The trip begins along a line of fencing in an area of old brick mill buildings, crosses **Center St.** a few blocks from downtown Southington, then parallels **South Center St.** in the shadow of a restored factory building.

Just ahead, trail travelers should use caution where the rail line diagonally crosses the busy intersection of **West Center St.** and **Bristol St.** Stop signs halt the car traffic and crosswalks lead across all four roads.

The setting remains industrial until the trail crosses a wooden bridge over the **Quinnipiac River** 0.7 miles south of the Mill St. parking lot. Benches invite a rest at this point and plenty of trees shelter the trail from surrounding signs of civilization. A narrow greenspace continues southward through a mixed residential and commercial neighborhood and the trail joins the shoulder of **Summer St.** before reaching **West Main St.** (1.3 miles) at the village of **Plantsville**. A circle of benches and memorial mark this point.

The next mile of trail traverse more commercial and industrial locations with the crossing of a wooden bridge over **Eight Mile River** along the way. It passes under **Exit 29** ramps for **I-84** (2.3 miles), intersects **Burritt St.** (2.7 miles), then crosses a bridge over **Rte. 322** near the area of **Milldale**. The trail enters woods as it passes the **Canal St.** trailhead parking lot (3.2 miles) and soon ends at the Cheshire town line.

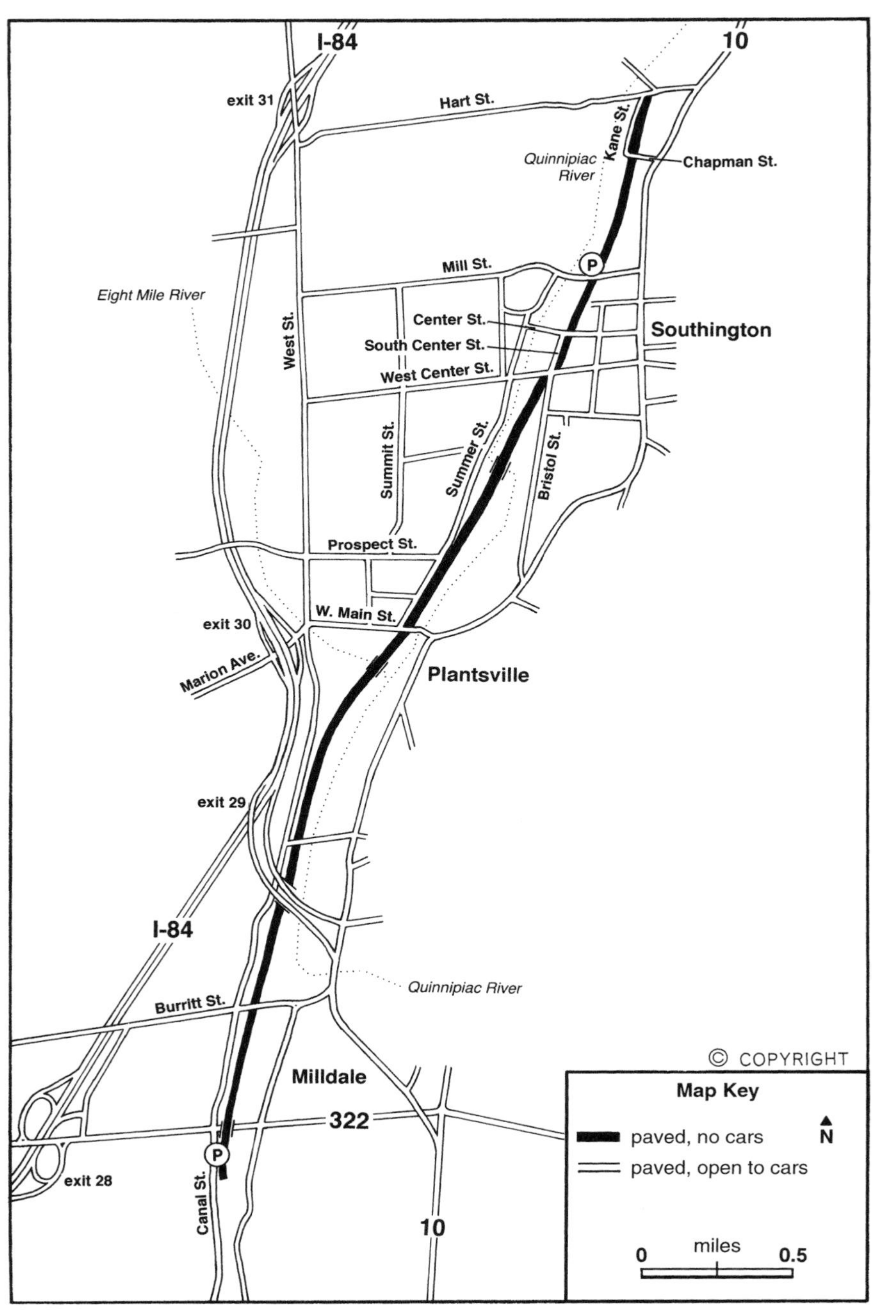
I-84
10
exit 31
Hart St.
Kane St.
Chapman St.
Quinnipiac River
Mill St.
Eight Mile River
West St.
Center St.
South Center St.
West Center St.
Southington
Summit St.
Summer St.
Bristol St.
Prospect St.
W. Main St.
exit 30
Marion Ave.
Plantsville
exit 29
I-84
Quinnipiac River
Burritt St.
Milldale
322
exit 28
Canal St.
10
© COPYRIGHT
Map Key
paved, no cars
paved, open to cars
N
miles
0
0.5

BACKGROUND:

The greenway follows the route of a former canal which was completed between New Haven and Farmington in 1828 and extended to Northampton, MA in 1836 to facilitate commerce between the seaport and the interior countryside. Measuring over 80 miles in length, it was the longest canal ever built in New England and one of the most complex requiring 28 locks to meet changes in elevation, 13 culverts to allow streams to flow beneath the canal, 3 aqueducts to carry the canal over rivers, and 135 bridges for local roads. The canal struggled to generate adequate revenues to repay these costs and closed in 1848 when a railroad began operation along the same route.

When the railroad ceased operation the route lay dormant for years. In the mid-1990's after the town of Cheshire built its rail-trail, Southington officials realized the line's potential as a linear parkland and in 2003 began construction of the northern half of this segment. The southern half was completed several years later. Future trail construction could include a short northward extension toward Plainville and completion of the trail in Cheshire to link the southern leg of the Greenway which extends to New Haven.

DRIVING DIRECTIONS:

Mill St. trailhead from I-84 southbound: Take Exit 32 and follow Rte. 10 south toward Southington. After 2 miles, turn right on Mill St. and look for the parking lot a short distance ahead on the right at the crossing of the trail.

Mill St. trailhead from I-84 northbound: Take Exit 30. Turn east (toward Southington) on Marion Ave. which becomes West Main St. at the next intersection. Continue to the end at Rte. 10 (Main St.), fork left (north) and follow Rte. 10 for 1.6 miles, then turn left on Mill St. Look for the trail-head parking lot a short distance ahead on the right at the crossing of the trail.

Canal St. trailhead from I-84: Take Exit 28 and follow Rte. 322 east for a half-mile. Turn right on Canal St. (just before passing under the rail-trail's bridge) and park ahead on the left.

TOILETS:

none on-site

ADDITIONAL INFORMATION:

Southington Parks Dept., (860) 276-6219

18 Farmington Valley Greenway Southwick Rail Trail

Farmington, CT - Southwick, MA

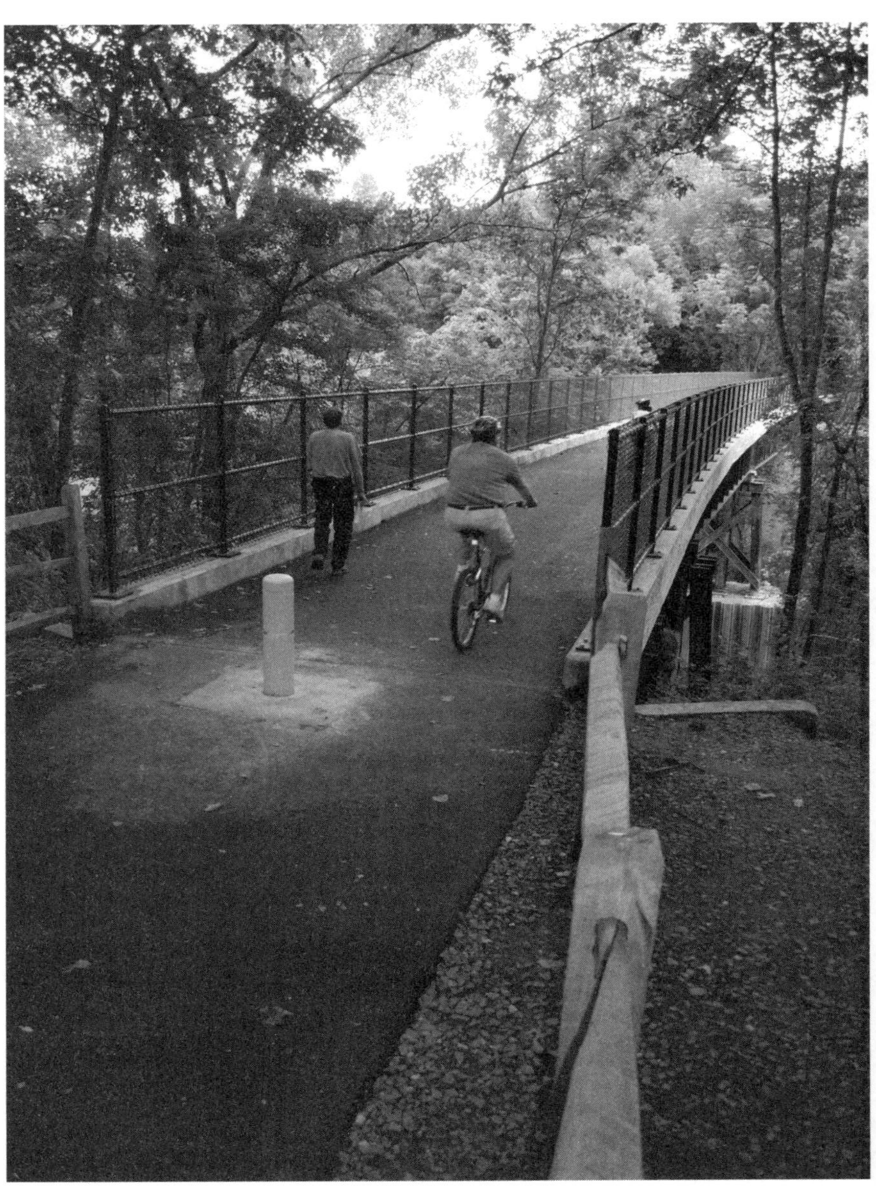

LENGTH: 28.7 miles
SURFACE: paved
TERRAIN: slight slopes, with hilly detours from rail line

Connecticut's grandest bike path, this section of the Farmington Greenway is a scenic marathon of villages, farmland, forests, and rivers. The trail joins six towns in two states with car-free commuting and recreation.

RULES & SAFETY:

- Bicyclists should yield to pedestrians.
- Keep to the right, pass on the left, and alert others (*"On your left..."*) when approaching from behind.
- Ride at a safe speed. The trail can be busy with walkers, runners, in-line skaters, and bicyclists so stay alert.
- Be especially careful in crowded areas, and in the presence of children and pets since their movements can be unpredictable.
- At road intersections, stop and look both ways when crossing and assume that drivers do not see you.
- Dogs must be leashed and their wastes removed.
- Keep the trail clean by caring out all that you carry in.
- When parking, be careful not to block trailhead gates and avoid leaving valuables inside your car.
- The area is open from sunrise to sunset.
- Since each town has its own set of policies for the trail, notice trailhead signs with additional regulations.

ORIENTATION:

This northernmost leg of the Farmington Greenway is an especially long route so plan your trip length carefully. It extends from Red Oak Hill Rd. in Farmington northward across the state line to join the Southwick Rail Trail in Southwick, MA. Scenery is good along the entire length but noticeably more rural along the northern half where large areas of woods and farmland surround the trail and fewer roads intersect it.

The trail encounters mild slopes along the route of the original canal and railroad, with low points near river and

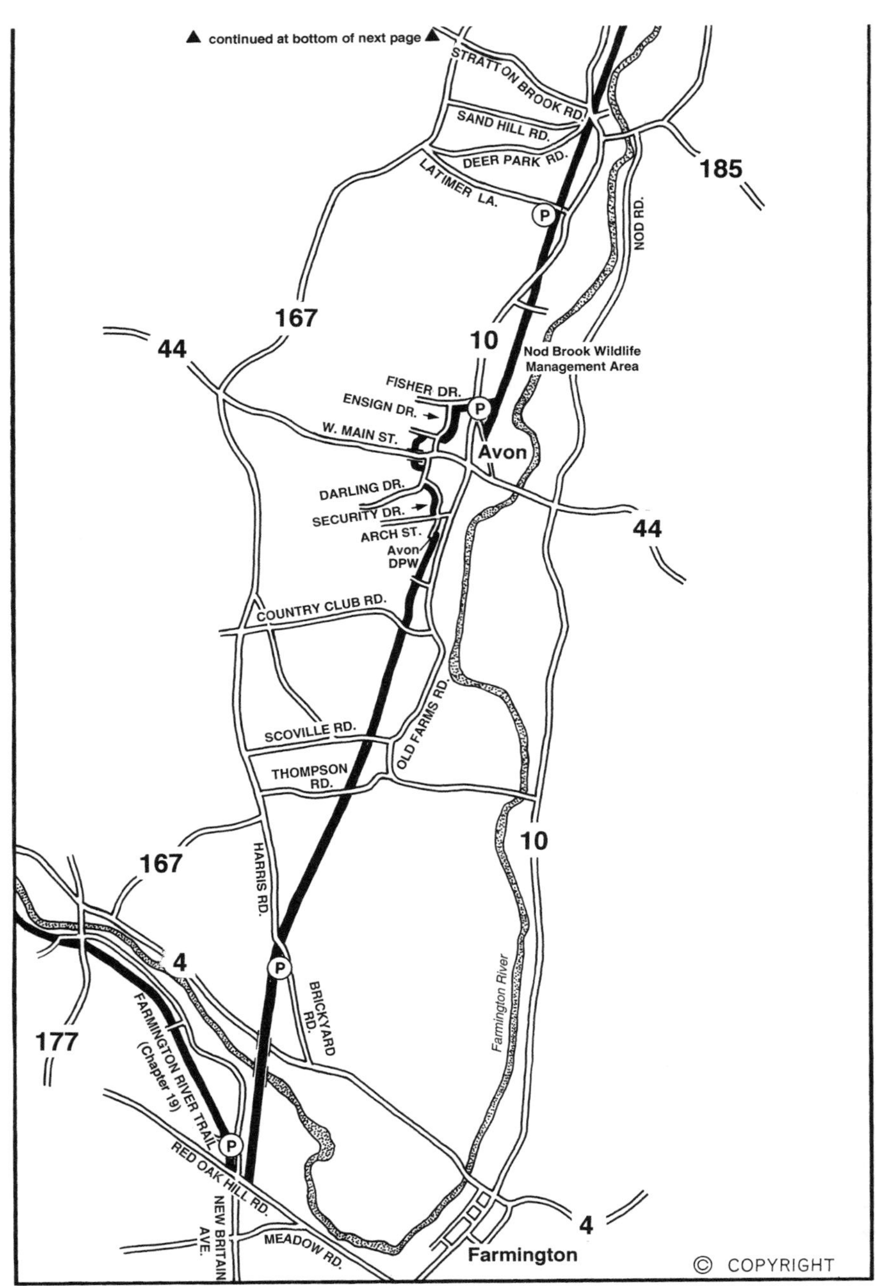

▲ continued at bottom of next page ▲
STRATTON BROOK RD.
SAND HILL RD.
DEER PARK RD.
LATIMER LA.
185
NOD RD.
167
44
10
Nod Brook Wildlife Management Area
FISHER DR.
ENSIGN DR.
W. MAIN ST.
Avon
DARLING DR.
SECURITY DR.
ARCH ST.
Avon DPW
44
COUNTRY CLUB RD.
OLD FARMS RD.
SCOVILLE RD.
THOMPSON RD.
10
167
HARRIS RD.
4
BRICKYARD RD.
Farmington River
177
FARMINGTON RIVER TRAIL (Chapter 19)
RED OAK HILL RD.
NEW BRITAIN AVE.
MEADOW RD.
4
Farmington
© COPYRIGHT

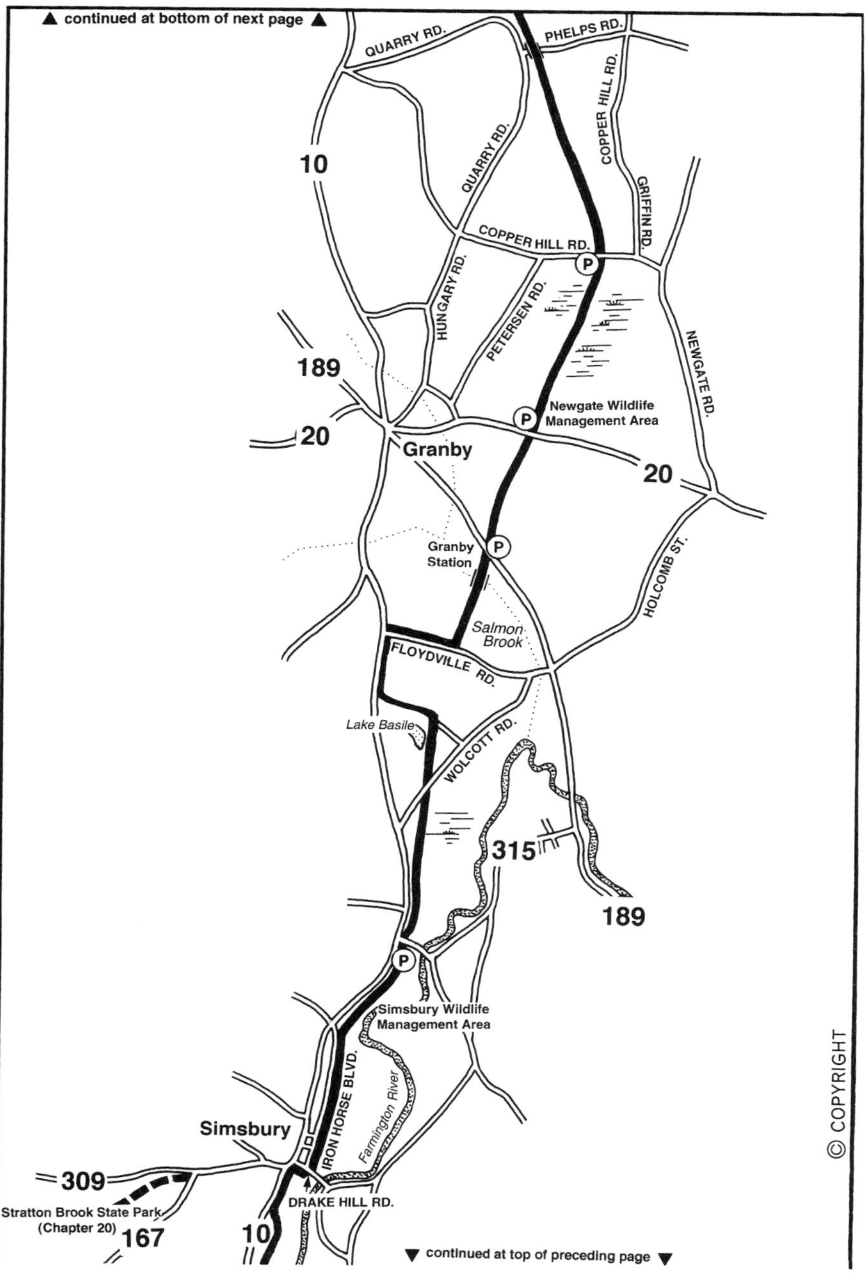
▲ continued at bottom of next page ▲
QUARRY RD.
PHELPS RD.
COPPER HILL RD.
10
QUARRY RD.
GRIFFIN RD.
COPPER HILL RD.
HUNGARY RD.
PETERSEN RD.
NEWGATE RD.
189
Newgate Wildlife
Management Area
20
Granby
20
Granby
Station
HOLCOMB ST.
Salmon
Brook
FLOYDVILLE RD.
Lake Basile
WOLCOTT RD.
315
189
Simsbury Wildlife
Management Area
IRON HORSE BLVD.
Farmington River
Simsbury
309
DRAKE HILL RD.
Stratton Brook State Park
(Chapter 20)
167
10
▼ continued at top of preceding page ▼
© COPYRIGHT

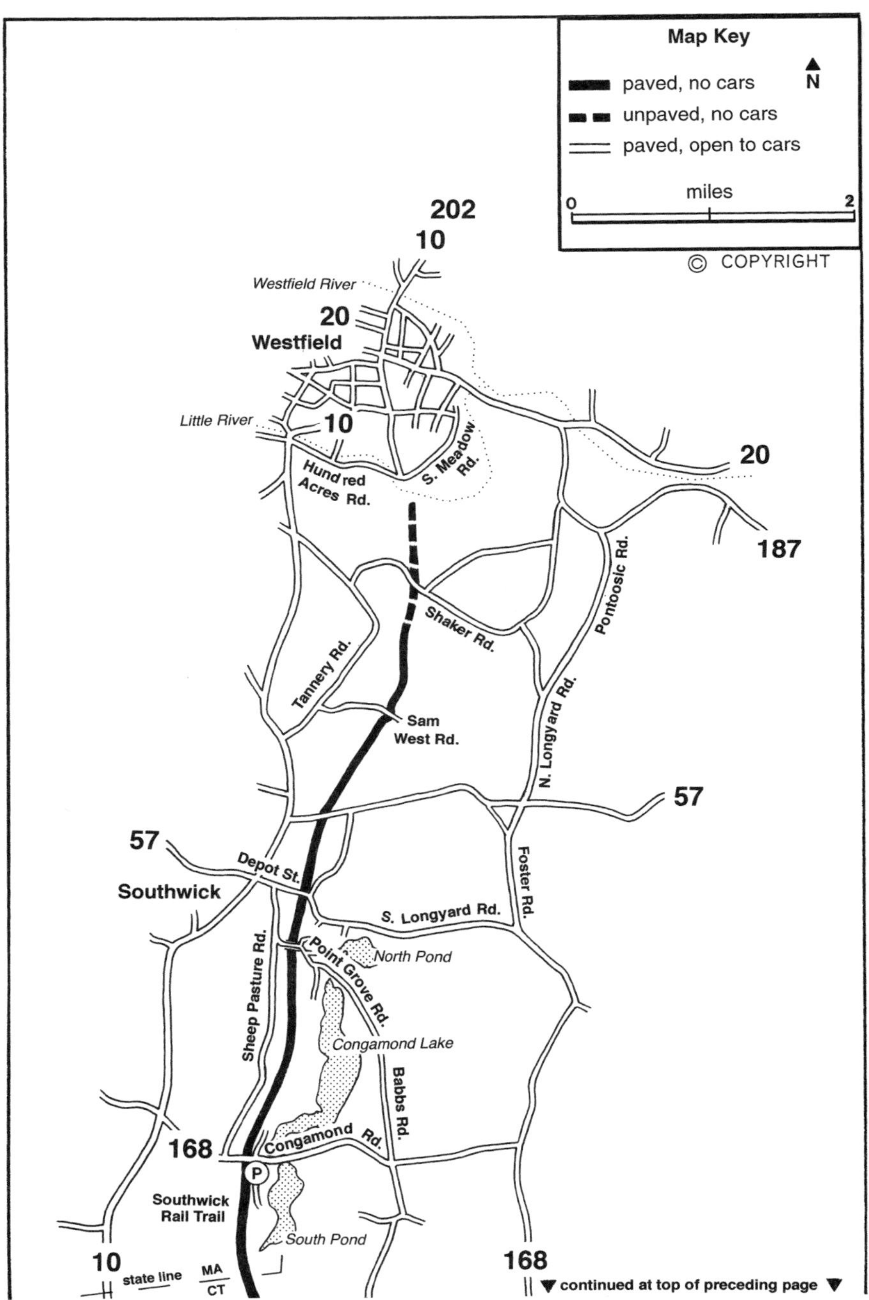

▼ continued at top of preceding page ▼

stream crossings and higher elevations in between. Bigger slopes exist where the trail detours from the rail line at the centers of Avon and Simsbury, as well as a few other locations. Note that the Avon detour also utilizes local roads at several points instead of a separated pathway.

Mileage markers posted beside the trail originate at Red Oak Hill Rd. in Farmington, the southern terminus. The trail has borders of mowed grass, protective fencing where necessary, and signs, crosswalks, and barricades to prevent vehicle entry at road intersections. Only the large trailheads are shown on the accompanying map and smaller parking areas exist at many trail/road intersections.

TRAIL DESCRIPTION:

Begin at the **Brickyard Rd.** trailhead in Farmington near the trail's southern endpoint. To the south (left), the trail runs for 2 miles to the terminus at **Red Oak Hill Rd.** with bridges spanning busy **Rte. 4** and a spectacular crossing of the **Farmington River** near the midpoint. At the end, turn right on Red Oak Hill Rd. to reach the nearby **Farmington River Tr.** (Chapter 19) located next to **New Britain Ave.**

Heading north (right) from the Brickyard Rd. trailhead, the paved trail extends for 26.7 miles. The trip starts on a straightaway with a faint downhill slope past the Avon town line, crosses **Thompson Rd.** after 1.5 miles, then enters the shade of woods for a half-mile. Open sky returns after **Scoville Rd.** (2.0 miles) where the trail straightens on a slight downhill along a line of telephone poles for a mile to **Country Club Rd.** (3.0 miles).

The trail leaves the rail bed as it approaches **Avon** center 3.7 miles north of the Brickyard Rd. trailhead and begins a 1.8-mile detour on a combination of local roads and separated pathway. Green *Bike Route* signs mark the way. Turning left at the end of the paved rail bed, the detour route joins the **Avon DPW** driveway and follows it north to **Arch St.**, then crosses the road and continues on a separated pathway beside **Security Dr.** After climbing a long slope, the route turns right on **Darling Dr.** and descends to another separated pathway which enters woods on the left side at the bottom of a slope and drops to a tunnel beneath **Rte. 44** (**W. Main St.**). Emerging at the police station on the other side, the route follows signs marking a right turn on **Climax**

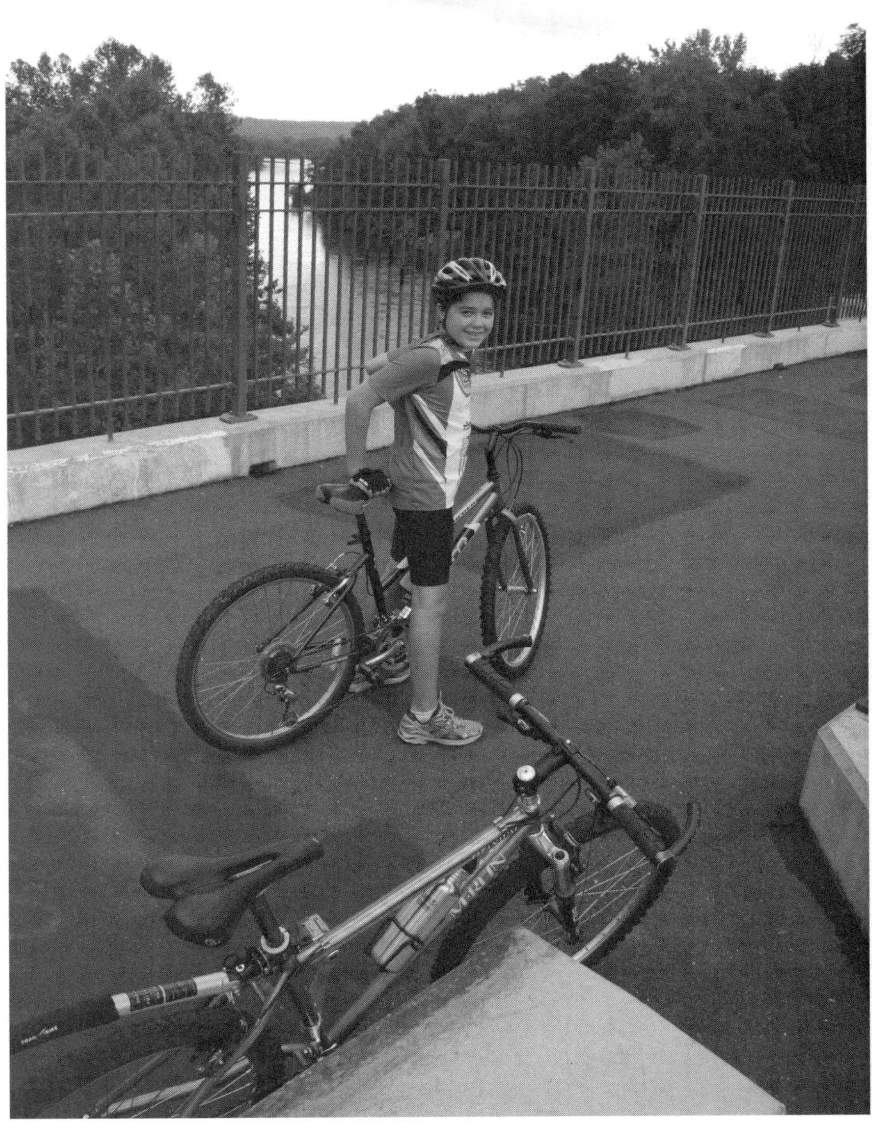

Heights Rd., left on a separated pathway beside **Ensign Dr.**, and then right at **Fisher Dr.** A crosswalk with signal at **Rte. 10** brings the trail past a trailhead and back to the rail bed (5.5 miles), where the greenway continues to the left (north). A short, dead end spur runs to the right (south) for 0.2 miles.

Continuing northward, the trail passes the **Nod Brook Wildlife Management Area** which preserves green space along the Farmington River on the right, then enters Simsbury and hits a number of road intersections. The busiest is another crossing of Rte. 10 (6.6 miles) about a mile beyond the Avon detour where heavy traffic deserves extra caution.

The greenway's next 1.3 miles follow another line of telephone poles past a trailhead parking lot at **Latimer La.** (7.0 miles), dipping at a few low points where wooden fencing corrals the trail across wetlands. It returns to Rte.10 at **Stratton Brook Rd.** (7.8 miles), crosses the busy intersection, and follows the edge of a parking lot on the other side.

Descending faintly, the trail takes a straight line course for almost a mile then turns sharply left and begins a second detour off the rail bed. It curves uphill for a quarter-mile to the side of Rte. 10, turns north along the edge of the road, and turns right alongside **Drake Hill Rd.** (9.6 miles). After a short descent, the greenway turns left (north) to cross the road at **Iron Horse Blvd.** (9.7 miles).

Returning to the original rail line, the trail follows a wooden guardrail separating Iron Horse Blvd. for a mile behind the commercial area of downtown **Simsbury**, then returns to the shade of woods for another mile surrounded by a broad swathe of grass and the preserved scenery of the **Simsbury Wildlife Management Area**. An overlook allows a view of the nearby Farmington River. The trail then merges at the foot of an embankment below Rte. 10, passes a trailhead, and intersects **Rte. 315** (11.7 miles).

The trail's remaining miles offer quieter surroundings

of woods and farmland. After passing another commercial area, the trail descends to a wetland along the river, intersects **Wolcott Rd.** (12.8 miles), and hits the East Granby town line near **Lake Basile**. It then makes a 1.7-mile detour around a plant nursery: turning left (west) off the rail bed, the trail follows a fence to Rte. 10 and continues as a separated pathway north to **Floydville Rd.** and then east back to the rail bed (15.0 miles) on the left after a half-mile.

Returning to forest shade, the trail crosses a high, curved bridge over **Salmon Brook** after a half-mile and soon reaches the former **Granby Station** house at **Rte. 189** (15.8 miles). It gains a slight incline for the next mile of woodsy surroundings to the intersection of **Rte. 20** (16.8 miles) at the parking lot for the **Newgate Wildlife Management Area** and, on the other side, continues gently uphill before flattening on a straight line through a wooded swamp.

North of **Copper Hill Rd.** (18.4 miles), the trail emerges in more open surroundings of farm fields and wetlands which allow distant views. After entering Suffield, it crosses a bridge over **Phelps Rd.** (20.1 miles), passes over two streams, then reaches the Massachusetts **state line** (20.5 miles) at a prominent granite post.

Here the trail enters the town of Southwick and becomes the **Southwick Rail Trail**. It continues beside a section of the old canal, cuts across an open wetland, and reaches **Congamond Rd.** (21.7 miles) near **Congamond Lake**, which is not visible. The trail rises on a noticeable slope past more farmland as it approaches Southwick center, then enters a tunnel under **Point Grove Rd.** (23.6 miles), intersects **Depot St.** a half-mile beyond, and crosses busy **Rte. 57** (24.8 miles) at a crosswalk and signal.

It enjoys a slight downslope for most of its remaining distance. The trail makes a straight line across a vast farm field, climbs and descends a banking at **Sam West Rd.** (25.9 miles), then ends at the Westfield city line, 26.7 miles north of the Brickyard Rd. trailhead. An unpaved trail continues along the rail bed for another 1.1 miles to the **Little River**.

BACKGROUND:

The greenway follows the route of a former canal which was completed between New Haven and Northampton, MA in 1836 to facilitate commerce between the seaport and the interior countryside. Measuring over 80 miles in length, it was the longest canal ever built in New England and one of the most complex requiring 28 locks to meet changes in elevation, 13 culverts to allow streams to flow beneath the canal, 3 aqueducts to carry the canal over rivers, and 135 bridges for roads. The canal struggled to generate adequate revenues to repay these costs and closed in 1848 when a railroad began operation along the same route.

After the railroad ceased using the tracks in 1988, local citizens formed the Farmington Valley Trails Council in 1992 to promote the creation of a recreational trail. Construction started in 1994 after federal funding was secured and it has progressed in phases since that time. The Farmington Valley Greenway joins other segments of this historic route (chapters 16 and 17) to form the Farmington Canal Heritage Trail which, with proposed future construction, will once again link New Haven and Northampton. The trail also forms a link in the East Coast Greenway which stretches from Maine to Florida.

DRIVING DIRECTIONS:

• **Brickyard Rd. trailhead, Farmington:** From I-84 take Exit 39 and follow Rte. 4 west for 2.7 miles. Turn right on Brickyard Rd. and park in the lot 1 mile ahead on the left.

• **Latimer La. trailhead, Simsbury:** From I-84 take Exit 50 and follow Rte. 44 west for 9.5 miles. Turn right on Rte. 10 north and continue for 2.2 miles, then turn left on Latimer La. and find the parking lot ahead on the left.

• **Rte. 10/Rte. 315 trailhead, Simsbury:** From I-91 take Exit 40 and follow Rte. 20 west for 9.4 miles to Granby. Turn left on Rte. 10 south and drive for 4.3 miles, then look for the trailhead on the left after the intersection of Rte. 315.

• **Rte. 20 trailhead, East Granby:** From I-91 take Exit 40 and follow Rte. 20 west for 8.2 miles. Park in the lot at the Newgate Wildlife Management Area where the trail crosses the road.

TOILETS:

in season at Thompson Rd. in Avon, Iron Horse Blvd. in Simsbury, Copper Hill Rd. in Suffield

ADDITIONAL INFORMATION:

Farmington Valley Trails Council, www.fvgreenway.org

19 Farmington River Trail

Farmington - Canton, CT

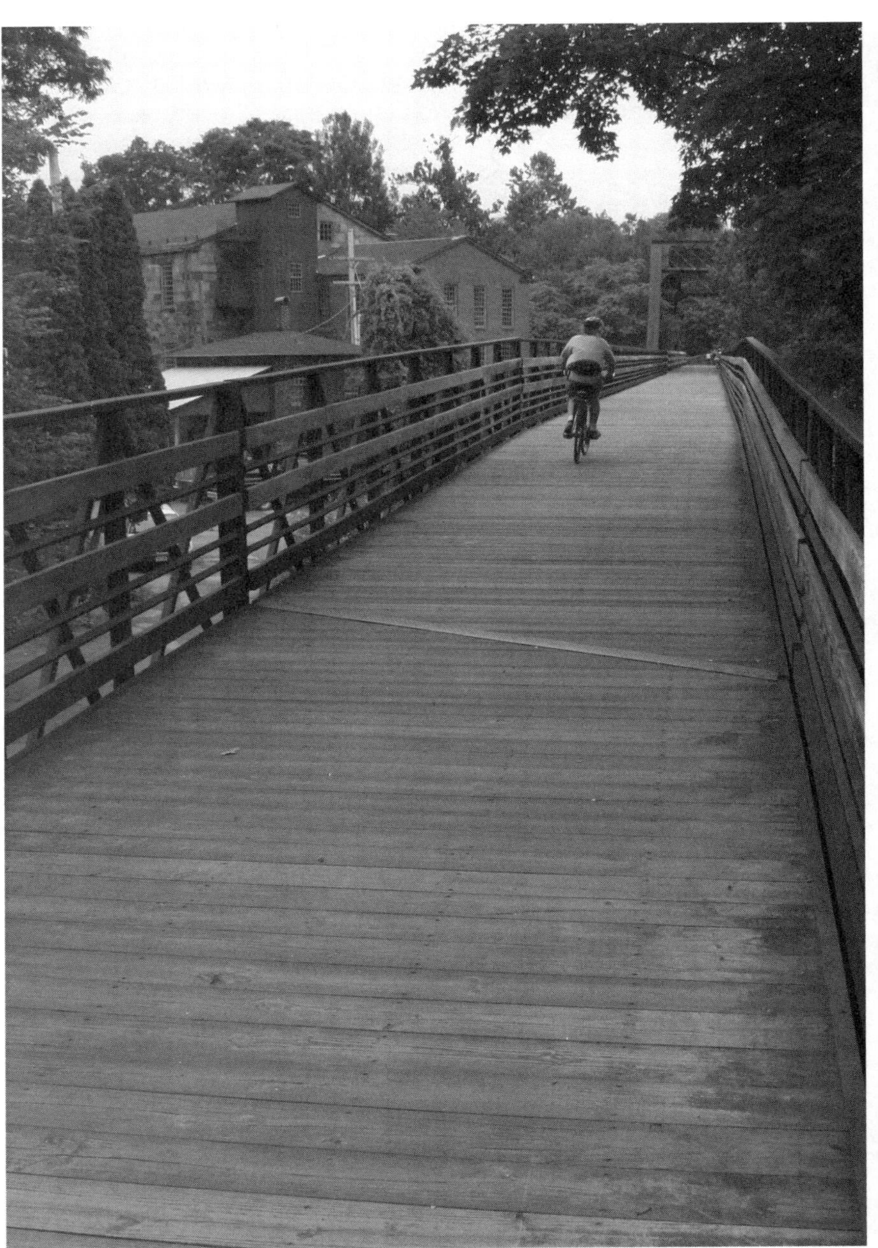

LENGTH: 10.2 miles
SURFACE: paved
TERRAIN: gentle slopes

Excellent scenery along the rapids of the Farmington River keeps this newly expanded rail-trail flowing with self-propelled traffic.

RULES & SAFETY:

- Bicyclists should yield to pedestrians.
- Keep to the right, pass on the left, and alert others (*"On your left..."*) when approaching from behind.
- Ride at a safe speed. Be especially cautious in crowded areas and when children or pets are present since their movements can be unpredictable.
- Step off the trail when stopped to allow others to pass.
- Stop at road intersections and assume that drivers do not see you.
- Respect the private property along the trail.
- Dogs must be leashed and their wastes removed.
- The trail is open from dawn until dusk.

ORIENTATION:

The Farmington River Trail extends in a mostly north-south direction from the intersection of Red Oak Hill Rd. and New Britain Ave. in Farmington (near the southern terminus of the Farmington Valley Greenway, detailed in Chapter 18) through Burlington to the intersection of Rte. 44 and Rte. 177 in Canton. Scenery is good along the entire trail length but is best along the midsection where it follows the banks of the Farmington River between the villages of Unionville and Collinsville.

Much of the paved surface is new but an older section of the trail in Burlington has become rippled by roots from surrounding trees and suffers from a bumpy ride as a result.

Wood fencing protects the trail at steep bankings, crosswalks and signs are in place at road intersections, and mileage markers provide distances from Red Oak Hill Rd. (the southern terminus) at half-mile intervals. Trailhead

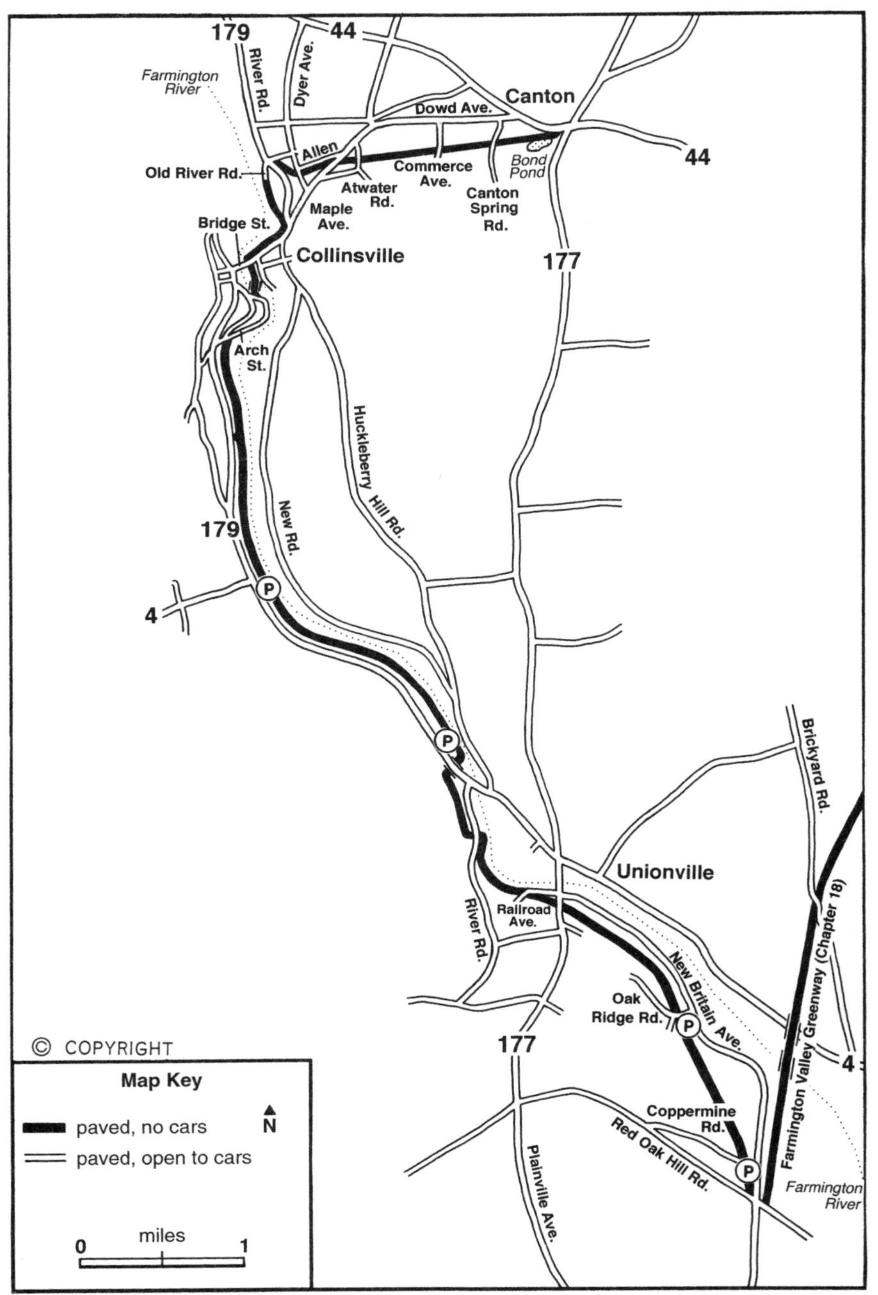
179
44
Farmington River
River Rd.
Dyer Ave.
Canton
Dowd Ave.
Allen
44
Old River Rd.
Commerce Ave.
Bond Pond
Atwater Rd.
Maple Ave.
Canton Spring Rd.
Bridge St.
Collinsville
177
Arch St.
Huckleberry Hill Rd.
New Rd.
179
4
Brickyard Rd.
Unionville
River Rd.
Railroad Ave.
Farmington Valley Greenway (Chapter 18)
New Britain Ave.
Oak Ridge Rd.
177
4
Coppermine Rd.
Red Oak Hill Rd.
Plainville Ave.
Farmington River
© COPYRIGHT
Map Key
paved, no cars
paved, open to cars
N
miles
0
1

parking lots exist at numerous points with the most popular ones being along the southern end of the trail. Note that the trail utilizes public roads (open to cars) for short distances at two points, but traffic is light along each.

TRAIL DESCRIPTION:

Beginning at the southernmost trailhead parking lot at **Copper Mine Rd.** and **New Britain Ave.** in Farmington, the trail extends in two directions. Turning left (south), it lasts for 0.2 miles to **Red Oak Hill Rd.** only a short distance from the southern end of the 28.7-mile **Farmington Valley Greenway**. (To reach it, cross New Britain Ave. heading east on Red Oak Hill Rd. and look for the greenway immediately ahead on the left.)

Turning right (north) on the Farmington River Trail, the trip starts in a mix of residential neighborhoods and wooded areas with a slight incline for the first half-mile. The slope tilts downward as the trail passes a second trailhead parking lot at the intersection of **Oak Ridge Rd.** (1.0 mile) and the downward angle lasts for the next mile to the outskirts of **Unionville** where it emerges at several depots and other railroad-era buildings. Wood fencing corrals the trail along a tight passageway at this point to the intersection of **Rte. 177** (**Plainville Ave.**) (2.1 miles).

After crossing this busy roadway, the trail soon intersects the end of **Railroad Ave.** and returns to natural scenery, this time along the west bank of the **Farmington River**. It passes a few homes in the area of **River Rd.** (2.2 miles) and then dips through a tunnel under **Rte. 4** (3.3 miles) where cylists should use caution since sharp turns limit visibility from both directions. A trailhead parking lot is located on the other side.

The next 3 miles are free of road intersections and, although parallel Rte. 4 is close, a slope separates the busy roadway so the trail offers enjoyable scenery in woods beside the river's rapids. The trail enters Burlington along the next mile and continues upstream along a narrow strip of land between the road and the river with a faint uphill grade.

After reaching a trailhead parking lot at the junction of **Rte. 179** (5.0 miles), the trail contends with a bumpy surface from tree roots in places. It crosses wooden bridges built across 3 streams along the next mile, and passes an old dam which creates a small waterfall on the river.

The separated path is interrupted at **Arch St.** (6.7 miles) where a 0.4-mile on-road detour begins. Turn right on Arch St. and continue upstream along the river past several homes, then look for the trail resuming at a wooden ramp on the right side. It rises to a trestle bridge over the Farmington River at the Canton town line and the edge of **Collinsville**, a mill village known for its manufacturing of knives, axes, and other metal edged products. Several signs sit beside the trail's next half-mile with historical information and photographs of the area.

Descending this high bridge on another ramp, the trail passes a cluster of mill buildings and a former railroad depot on the way to the intersection of **Bridge St.** (**Rte. 179**) (7.4 miles). Turning right, it parallels the road for the next third of a mile, separates at a wooden deck built along the river, crosses a bridge over Rattlesnake Brook, and passes behind a sewage treatment plant to reach the end of **Old River Rd.** (8.1 miles) where a second on-road leg begins. Follow the road for a short distance to Rte. 179 and cross carefully to continue on the next section of trail.

It begins with an uphill slope to **Dyer Ave.** (8.4 miles) and then flattens alongside **Allen Place** to the intersection of busy **Maple Ave.** (8.7 miles), where caution is required when crossing.

The trail continues across another bridge over Rattlesnake Brook and the intersection of **Atwater Rd.** (8.8 miles), then straightens through a wooded area for the next mile intersecting **Commerce Ave.** (9.3 miles) and **Canton Spring Rd.** (9.6 miles) along the way. After passing **Bond Pond** on the right, the trail ends beside **Rte. 44** (Albany Tpke.) (10.0 miles) at the junction of **Rte. 177** near the center of Canton.

BACKGROUND:

The Farmington River Trail utilizes two former railroads along its 10-mile course. The southern end of the trail follows a railroad spur which was built off the New Haven and Northampton Railroad in 1850 to serve Unionville, Burlington, and the burgeoning manufacturing operations at Collinsville. North of Collinsville, the trail turns onto the former Connecticut Western Railroad which was built in 1871 between Hartford and the New York state line and provided an important transportation route for coal entering New England.

After the usefulness of these rail lines had passed, the state's Dept. of Transportation acquired the routes and transferred management to the Dept. of Environmental Protection in 1988 in order to enable the creation of the trail. Construction has progressed in numerous phases, with the first two segments of trail built in 1999 and 2000 and the most recent section completed in 2011. Additional work has been proposed.

DRIVING DIRECTIONS:

New Britain Ave. trailhead from I-84 northbound: Take Exit 33 and follow Rte. 72 west, then take Exit 1 and follow Rte. 177 north for 2.9 miles. Turn right (east) on Meadow Rd. and drive for 1 mile, then turn left (north) on New Britain Ave. and continue for 0.7 miles to the trailhead on the left.

New Britain Ave. trailhead from I-84 southbound: Take Exit 39 for Rte. 4 west. At the first traffic signal, measure 1 mile on Rte. 4 west, then turn left on Rte. 10 south and proceed for 0.9 miles. Turn right (west) on Meadow Rd. and drive for 1 mile, keep straight on Red Oak Hill Rd. (where Meadow Rd. forks left) and continue for 0.7 miles, then turn right (north) on New Britain Ave. The trailhead is just ahead on the left.

Trailhead at junction of Rte. 4/Rte. 179: From I-84 take Exit 39 and follow Rte. 4 west for 8.3 miles. Look for the parking lot on the right at the traffic signal where Rte. 4 turns left and Rte. 179 continues straight.

TOILETS:

none on-site

ADDITIONAL INFORMATION:

Farmington Valley Trails Council, www.fvgreenway.org

20 Stratton Brook State Park

Simsbury, CT

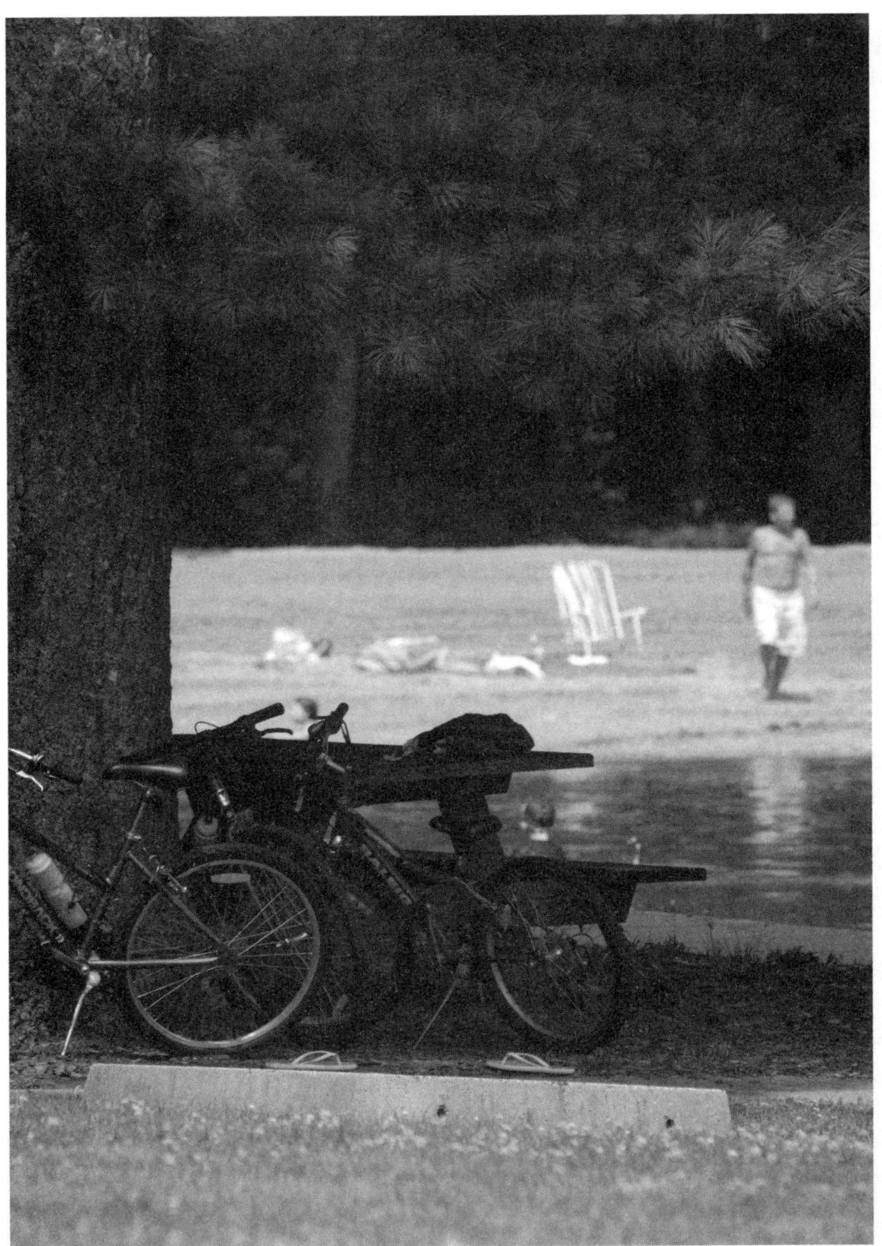

LENGTH: 3.3 miles, including 1.4-mile on-road section
SURFACE: stone dust
TERRAIN: flat

This small, family-friendly state park has something for everyone: a swimming beach, fishing hole, picnic area, and, for those who can't sit still, a pleasant stretch of rail-trail. Beware that it's a popular place on summer weekends.

RULES & SAFETY:

- Bicyclists must yield to pedestrians.
- Keep to the right, ride at a safe speed, and alert others (*"On your left..."*) when approaching from behind.
- Use extra caution in the area of the swimming and fishing ponds since it can be busy with people.
- Be especially careful when children and pets are present since their movements can be unpredictable.
- Horses and motorized vehicles are prohibited.
- An admission fee is charged when entering the park by car during the summer season.
- The area is open from 8:00 AM until sunset.

ORIENTATION:

The rail-trail has a northeast-southwest alignment and stretches for 3.3 miles from end to end. It exists in two separate segments which are joined by a 1.4-mile section of Town Forest Rd., a public road which is open to cars. Car traffic is typically light. Stratton Brook State Park lies along the longer, northeast leg of the trail where trail usage is highest. The shorter southwest leg gets noticeably less use.

The trail's stone dust surface is firm, smooth, and about 10 feet wide. Gates block vehicle entry at road intersections, which are few.

TRAIL DESCRIPTION:

From **Stratton Brook State Park**, turn left on the rail-trail and follow it in the northeasterly direction toward Simsbury for a mile-long trip (one way). The trail leaves the lively area of the swimming and fishing ponds and immediately enters the peace and quiet of evergreen forest,

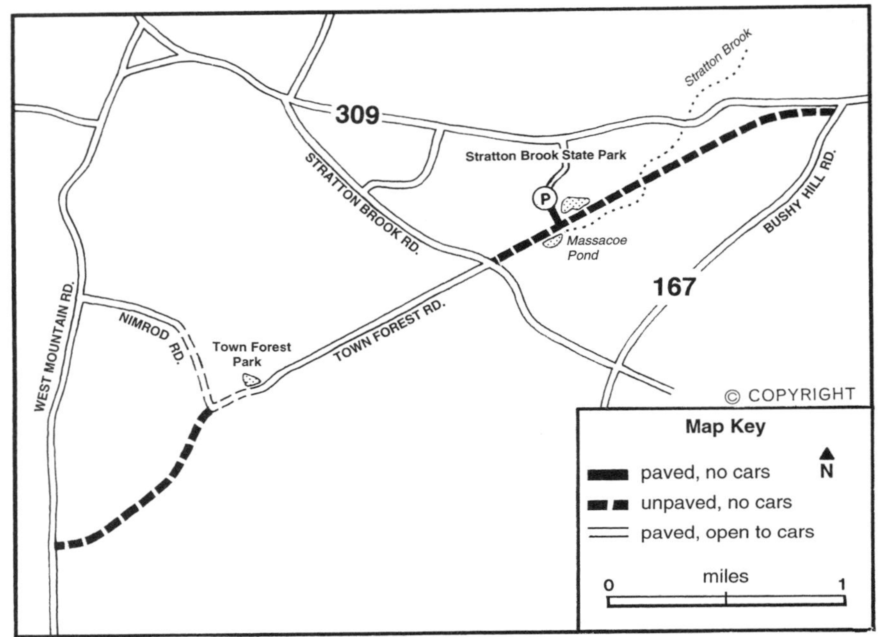

crossing a bridge over **Stratton Brook** after a third of a mile. Tall trees stand close to the surface providing shade from summer heat and a natural feel to the ride. After three quarters of a mile, the straight-line course gives way to a gentle right-hand curve just before the trail ends at **Bushy Hill Rd.** (**Rte. 167**).

Heading in the opposite direction from the park's trail-head, the bike path ventures toward the southwest along the same straight corridor, leaving **Massacoe Pond** on a quarter-mile leg to the crossing of **Stratton Brook Rd.**

Continue straight on **Town Forest Rd.** for the next 1.4 miles to reach the next section of trail. This little-traveled road was built atop the railroad grade and its paved surface changes to gravel near the end at a sharp, right turn where **Nimrod Rd.** begins. The rail-trail goes straight at this intersection, rising on a slight slope beneath tall pines and passing between two residential neighborhoods on the final 0.7-mile leg before the end at **West Mountain Rd.**

BACKGROUND:

This trail follows the route of the Connecticut Western Railroad which was built in 1871 between Hartford and the New York state line. The railroad struggled with a rough topography and achieved only modest importance, although it carried a steady flow of coal into New England. Through service on the Connecticut Western ended in the early 1930's and most of the line fell idle by the 1960's. The area of Stratton Brook State Park, which was originally part of Massacoe State Forest, served as a testing area for minimizing the risk of forest fires caused by sparks from passing steam engines, a persistent problem at the time.

Train travel ceased on this section of the line during the Great Depression and the Civilian Conservation Corps (C.C.C.) pulled up the tracks in 1937 so that visitors to the newly formed state park could enjoy the route. The C.C.C. also dammed Stratton Brook to create a swimming pond which remains the park's main attraction. The rail-trail's surface was upgraded as a bike path in 1972 by the Simsbury Recreation Dept.

DRIVING DIRECTIONS:

From I-91 take Exit 40. Follow Rte. 20 west for 9.4 miles to Granby, then turn left on Rte. 10 south and continue for 6.4 miles to Simsbury. Turn right on Rte. 167 south and drive for 0.8 miles, then stay straight on Rte. 309 west and continue for another 0.9 miles to the park entrance on the left.

From I-84 take Exit 50. Follow Rte. 44 west for 9.5 miles, then turn right on Rte. 10 north and drive for 3.8 miles to Simsbury. Turn left on Rte. 167 south and continue for 0.8 miles, then stay straight on Rte. 309 west and continue for another 0.9 miles to the park entrance on the left.

TOILETS:

Stratton Brook State Park during the summer season

ADDITIONAL INFORMATION:

Stratton Brook State Park, c/o Penwood State Park, 57 Gun Mill Rd., Bloomfield, CT 06002, (860) 242-1158

21 MDC Nepaug Reservoir

Canton & Burlington, CT

LENGTH: 2 sections totaling 3 miles
SURFACE: paved
TERRAIN: one section is gentle, the other is hilly
NOTE: not recommended for in-line skating

These almost forgotten stretches of roadway along the Nepaug Reservoir are closed to car traffic and open for recreation. They are a smaller, quieter alternative to the Metropolitan District Commission's West Hartford facility (Chapter 22) and offer equally good scenery with numerous water views.

RULES & SAFETY:

- The MDC manages this water supply property with strict rules. Recreational use is limited to Torrington Ave. and Clear Brook Rd., and use of other roads is forbidden. Officers patrol the area to enforce the regulations.
- Bicyclists are required to wear helmets.
- Bicyclists should yield to pedestrians. Alert others (*"On your left..."*) when approaching from behind to avoid startling them.
- Dogs must be leashed and their wastes removed.
- Swimming and fishing are prohibited.
- Be careful not to block trailhead gates when parking since work crews and emergency vehicles need access.
- The area is open from dawn until dusk.

ORIENTATION:

Two paved, car-free roads are available for the public to use. Mile-long Torrington Ave. follows the reservoir's northern shoreline with mild slopes, smooth pavement, and several good views over the water. Two-mile Clear Brook Rd. follows the southern shoreline with hillier, rougher, and more isolated conditions. These two roads are separated by a very hilly, 2.5-mile on-road ride.

Note that the nearby Farmington River Tr. (Chapter 19) is located a few hundred feet in elevation below the reservoir, so a strenuous uphill effort is required when riding between the two locations.

Other than the metal gates blocking vehicle entry and the pavement itself, no amenities exist.

TRAIL DESCRIPTION:

Mile-long **Torrington Ave.** starts at **Rte. 202** with a view over a meadow to the **Nepaug Reservoir**. The road parallels the shoreline on a slope above the water, visible through woods, and offers a slight downhill grade for the 0.4 miles to **Nepaug Dam**, where it turns sharply right. The 600'-long crescent-shaped dam provides views both over the reservoir and down the spillway which drops 130' to the **Nepaug River**.

The road crosses the dam and enters woods on the other side. Rising on a gentle incline, it continues paralleling the shoreline at a distance while curving through forest, then reaches the eastern gate at the 1-mile mark. Here Torrington Ave. is open to car traffic and descends for 1.2 miles to the village of **Collinsville** and the **Farmington River Tr.** (Chapter 19).

Alone at the southern end of the reservoir, 2-mile **Clear Brook Rd.** has a more isolated feel and noticeably older pavement, with an abundance of potholes and cracks warranting caution from cyclists especially on slopes.

Beginning near **Barnes Hill Rd.** at the eastern end, the road immediately tilts downhill from the trailhead gate along a row of larch trees and old stone walls. After a quarter-mile it joins the reservoir's shoreline at the bottom, curves around a small cove, then straightens with relatively flat pedaling until the 1-mile mark where an uphill grade develops. The road approaches the sound of **Clear Brook** which it follows up a valley into the reservation's protected woodlands. The pitch steepens as it climbs beside the brook then moderates as the road turns southward and ends at a metal gate near the intersection of **Foote Rd.**

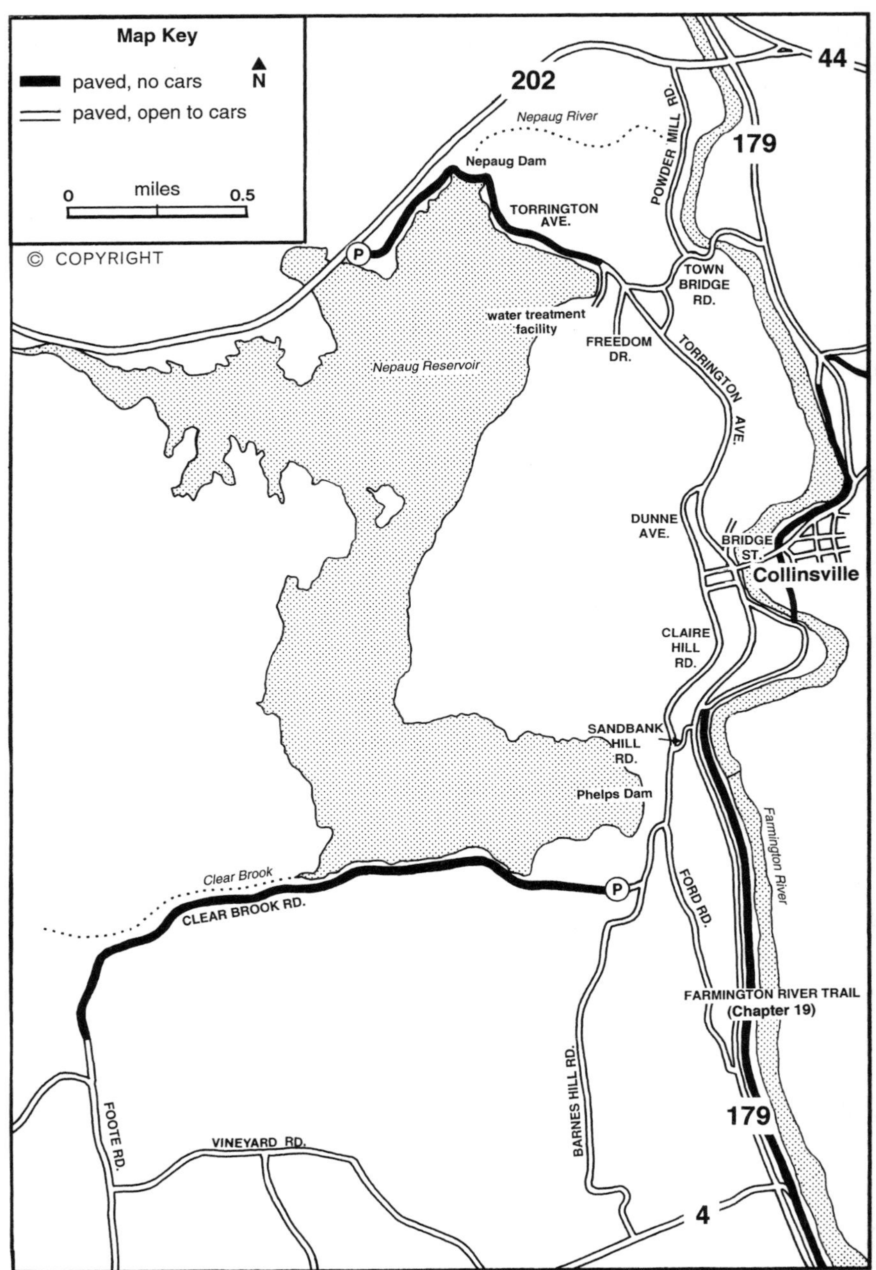
Map Key
paved, no cars
paved, open to cars
N
0
miles
0.5
© COPYRIGHT
202
44
179
Nepaug River
Nepaug Dam
POWDER MILL RD.
TORRINGTON AVE.
TOWN BRIDGE RD.
water treatment facility
FREEDOM DR.
TORRINGTON AVE.
Nepaug Reservoir
DUNNE AVE.
BRIDGE ST.
Collinsville
CLAIRE HILL RD.
SANDBANK HILL RD.
Phelps Dam
Farmington River
Clear Brook
CLEAR BROOK RD.
FORD RD.
FARMINGTON RIVER TRAIL (Chapter 19)
BARNES HILL RD.
FOOTE RD.
VINEYARD RD.
179
4

BACKGROUND:

A special act of the Connecticut General Assembly sparked the creation of the Nepaug Reservoir during the years 1911 to 1916. In order to expand Hartford's water supply system, the city's water authority purchased all of the properties in and around the flood zone and built two large dams to contain the reservoir. The village of Nepaug, a settlement of small farms dating from the late 1700's, was evacuated and its 22 houses, local school, and church were either relocated or destroyed. The graves of Nepaug's two cemeteries were moved to nearby Collinsville. At the time, the project ranked as the greatest engineering feat for a water supply in New England.

The tributary waters of the Nepaug River, Clear Brook, and Phelps Brook supply the reservoir with spring-fed run-off from the bordering hills.

DRIVING DIRECTIONS:

- **Torrington Ave. trailhead:** From I-84 take Exit 50 and follow Rte. 44 west for 15 miles. Turn left on Rte. 202 west and continue for 1.5 miles, then look for the trailhead on the left before the reservoir.
- **Clear Brook Rd. trailhead:** From I-84 take Exit 39 and follow signs for Rte. 4 west. From the next traffic signal, continue for 7.7 miles on Rte. 4 west to the junction of Rte. 179. Turn left and continue on Rte. 4 west for another half-mile, then turn right on Barnes Hill Rd. and drive for 1.3 miles. Turn left on Clear Brook Rd. and park near the gate being careful not to block access.

TOILETS:

none on-site

ADDITIONAL INFORMATION:

Metropolitan District Commission, P.O. Box 800, Hartford, CT 06142-0800, (860) 278-7850, www.themdc.com

22 MDC W. Hartford Reservoirs

West Hartford, CT

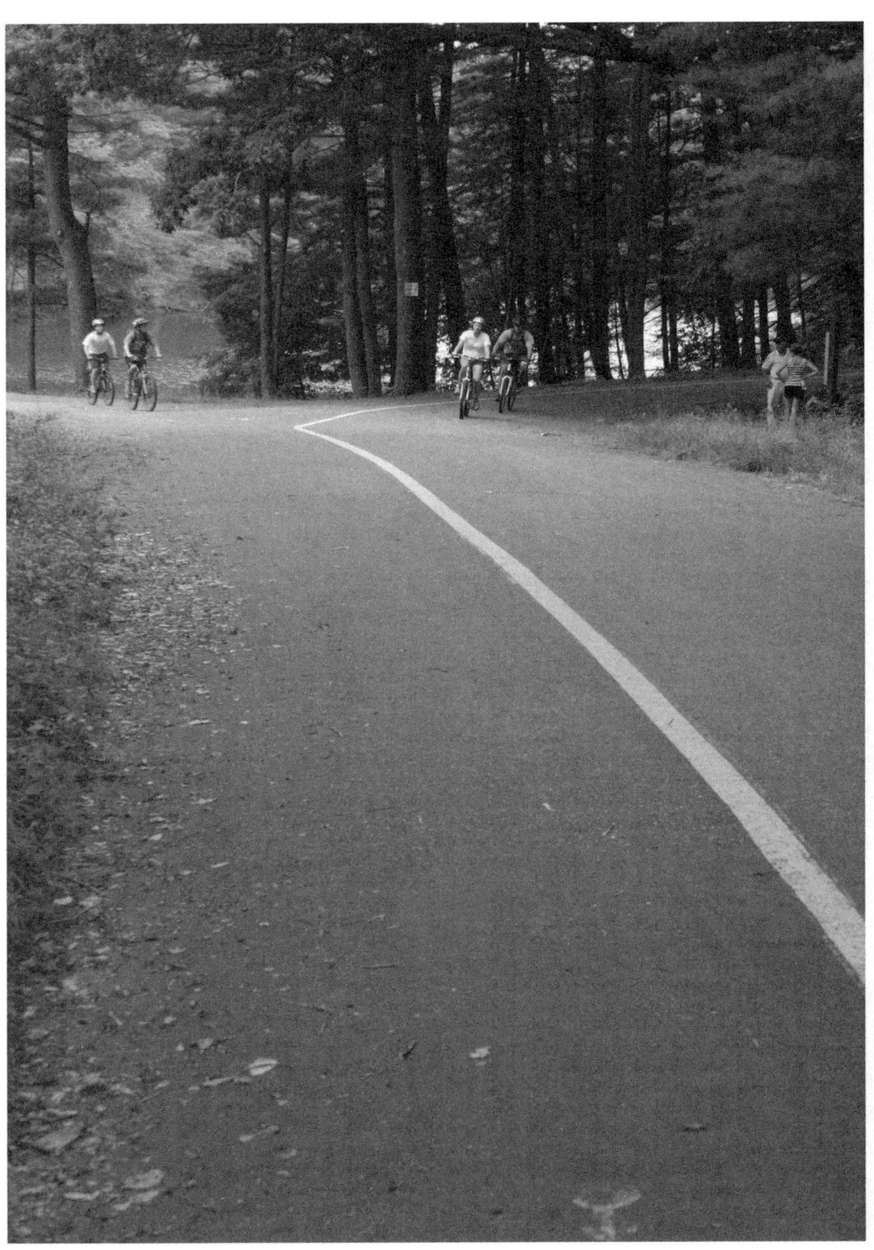

LENGTH: 13 miles
SURFACE: about half paved, half gravel
TERRAIN: varies from gently rolling to hilly

Greater Hartford's favorite playground, this 3,000-acre parkland is an oasis for bicyclists, mountain bikers, in-line skaters, walkers, and runners. The gated roads roll and curve through natural scenery of lakes and forest.

RULES & SAFETY:

• Bicyclists must wear helmets. In-line skaters must wear helmets as well as knee, elbow, and wrist protection.

• Bicyclists and in-line skaters are asked to be courteous to pedestrians, and to use the designated bike lane where it is present.

• Step out of the way when stopped so others can pass unimpeded.

• Use extra caution in crowded areas, and when children and pets are present since their movements can be unpredictable.

• Bicycling is not permitted on the bankings which line the many dams and impoundments, and on trails that are marked with signs reading *No Bikes*.

• Since this land serves as a water supply area, the MDC enforces strict rules (posted at trailheads) in order to protect the watershed. Swimming and fishing are among the prohibited activities.

• Dogs must be leashed and their wastes removed.

• The park is open from sunrise until either 8:00 PM or one half-hour after sunset, whichever is earlier.

• Watch for additional regulations posted at trailheads.

ORIENTATION:

An extensive network of gated roads, some paved and some unpaved, explores this vast property of reservoirs and woodlands. Display maps with *"You are here"* designations are stationed at a couple of points along the most heavily traveled routes but few other signs are present to guide newcomers. Bring a map of the area when visiting

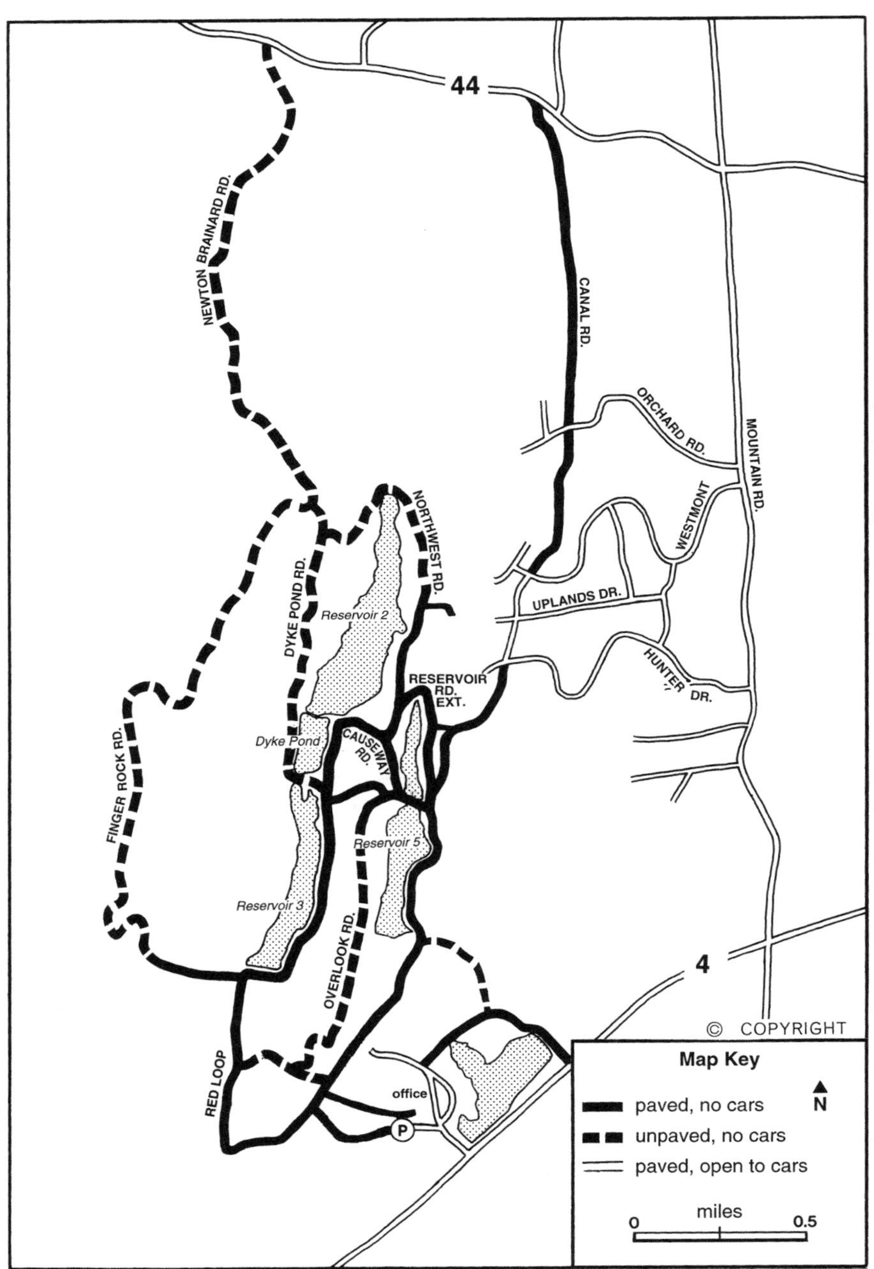

44
NEWTON BRAINARD RD.
CANAL RD.
ORCHARD RD.
MOUNTAIN RD.
NORTHWEST RD.
WESTMONT
DYKE POND RD.
Reservoir 2
UPLANDS DR.
HUNTER DR.
RESERVOIR RD. EXT.
FINGER ROCK RD.
Dyke Pond
CAUSEWAY RD.
Reservoir 5
Reservoir 3
OVERLOOK RD.
4
© COPYRIGHT
Map Key
paved, no cars
unpaved, no cars
paved, open to cars
N
miles
0
0.5
RED LOOP
office
P

for the first time and track your progress as you go.

The 6 miles of paved roads keep to gentler terrain in the area of the reservoirs and include a popular, 3.4-mile one-way loop which is identifiable by a bike lane painted on its surface. About 7 miles of unpaved roads venture farther into the woods and have less usage, bigger hills, fewer signs and navigational aids, and rough surfaces in several spots.

TRAIL DESCRIPTION:

Begin with the scenic, 3.4-mile **Red Loop** which offers a wide paved surface, a painted bike lane, and views of several reservoirs. To find it from the main trailhead, either continue past the gate at the end of the parking lot or follow the trail from the center of the parking lot over a bridge and then turn left along a fence. Both options end at the Red Loop (which is apparent from its painted bike lane), where bicyclists must turn left because it is designated for one-way travel in the clockwise direction.

The road starts with a hill climb, then turns northward at the top and flattens. Near the 1-mile mark it rises on a second slope to a dam containing **Reservoir 3**, circles the southern end of the reservoir and continues northward beside the shore. This stretch offers flat riding and intersects Middle Rd. and Dyke Pond Rd. along the way.

Red Loop turns eastward at **Reservoir 2** and encounters a series of small, rolling hills and numerous intersections. The painted bike lane guides riders through the choices, descending at first on **Causeway Rd.**, forking left onto **Northwest Rd.**, and turning right on **Reservoir Rd. Extension**. After circling the northern end of **Reservoir 5**, the loop returns southward past the end of Canal Rd. at the 2.6-mile mark and finishes with flat riding along Reservoir 5 with frequent views over the water.

Middle Rd. and Causeway Rd. bisect this loop with slightly shorter alternatives. Both roads descend toward the east and send riders across Reservoir 5 on an earthen causeway.

Lesser-traveled **Canal Rd.** offers a 2.3-mile spur with

a mostly flat course on the bed of a former canal, although a short distance along the midsection is open to cars. Heading northward from Reservoir 5, it starts with an uphill and then flattens with a curving route which slips through several residential neighborhoods on a narrow strip of public land. At the half-mile mark it is open to cars for a third of a mile but the traffic is very light. Car-free pavement resumes for the remaining 1.5 miles to busy **Rte. 44** (Albany Tpke.) where an abrupt drop to the roadway deserves extreme caution. Biking along this high speed, four-lane road is not recommended.

Gravel roads provide additional options although their hills tend to be larger and their surfaces can be rough in spots. **Overlook Rd.** occupies high ground above Reservoir 5 and requires a strenuous climb which is most gradual when ridden from north to south. Once on top, riders enjoy a mile of gently rolling terrain before they descend a steeper, rougher slope at the southern end of the road.

Finger Rock Rd. holds the biggest hills. It starts from Red Loop at the southern tip of Reservoir 3 and climbs in switchbacks for almost a mile on a surface that alternates between old pavement and gravel. The steepest points have washouts which are a hindrance for cyclists. After passing prominent rock outcroppings, the road flattens at its highest elevation with a smooth firm surface and passes Finger Rock, a formation of ledge which is easily noticed at the inside of a long, left-hand turn. At the northern end, the final 1.2 miles are a gradual downhill with a few parts being moderately steep and slightly eroded.

Two options continue from the northern terminus of Finger Rock Rd. **Newton Brainard Rd.** heads northward for 1.5 miles to Rte. 44 through rolling, forested terrain which includes one significant downhill with a loose surface near the 1-mile mark. Aside from the sight of a powerline and a gas pipeline, it offers purely natural surroundings in one of the more remote corners of the park.

Returning to the south, mile-long **Dyke Pond Rd.**

curves through an area of rock outcroppings before descending gradually along a slope to **Dyke Pond** and the pavement of Red Loop. Along the way it intersects **Northwest Rd.**, also a mile in length, which drops more quickly for a third of a mile, rounds the northern tip of Reservoir 2, and returns through gentle terrain to the paved routes.

BACKGROUND:

The Metropolitan District Commission (MDC) is a state-chartered organization which manages this property and others for Hartford's water supply and for passive recreation. This 3,000-acre tract has been used as a public water supply since 1867 and its trails, woods, and scenic water views have been drawing recreational visitors since that time. Today it is one of greater Hartford's largest open space areas and its network of gated roads and trails are a year-round attraction.

DRIVING DIRECTIONS:

From I-84 take Exit 39 (not Exit 39A for Rte. 4). At the first traffic signal, turn right on Rte. 4 east and drive for 2.3 miles to the park entrance, on the left. Fork left at the first intersection following signs for recreational parking.

TOILETS:

portable toilets at the start of the Red Loop

ADDITIONAL INFORMATION:

Metropolitan District Commission (MDC), P.O. Box 800, Hartford, CT 06142-0800, (860) 278-7850, www.themdc.com

23 Penwood State Park

Bloomfield

LENGTH: 3.7-mile loop
SURFACE: mostly old pavement, partly stone dust
TERRAIN: hilly
NOTE: not suited for in-line skating

The crumbling pavement of an old road clings to this quiet park's woodsy ridgeline with a fun loop for bicycling and the chance to enjoy distant views.

RULES & SAFETY:

• Bicyclists should yield to pedestrians.

• Alert others (*"On your left..."*) when approaching from behind to avoid startling them.

• Ride at a safe speed and keep to the right side. The many slopes and blind corners can be dangerous for two-way traffic.

• Be aware of the road's unique centerline drains which effectively shed rainwater but, resembling pot holes, present a hazard for bicycling.

• Note that the asphalt is aging and its cracks and bumps are sometimes obscurred by forest debris.

• The park is open during daylight hours.

ORIENTATION:

Penwood's distinctive topography assists visitors in tracking their location as the park's only road forms a long, slender loop around a north-south ridgeline. Few signs exist to guide visitors but few are needed since the road's pavement forms a self-contained loop with few opportunities for wrong turns.

Elevation changes are significant, with the road's highest point being near the Cedar Ridge Overlook and the lowest being at Shadow Pond. Two short sections of the loop share the park's road with cars (beside Gale Pond and near Shadow Pond), but traffic is minimal.

TRAIL DESCRIPTION:

Park Rd. forms a 3.7-mile loop through Penwood's dramatic terrain. The road ascends and descends sizeable hills and, for much of its distance, follows a shelf cut into the hillside where rock and ledge rise on one side and the slope falls away on the other.

Following the loop in the counter-clockwise direction from the **Gale Pond** trailhead parking lot beside **Rte. 185**, begin on the 1.3-mile access road to the ranger station. This narrow road is sometimes open to car traffic, posted with a 10 m.p.h. speed limit, and gets little use. Follow it along the boundary fence beside Gale Pond, first around a right-hand turn and then to a left-hand turn (at 0.2 miles). Fork right on an unpaved bike path at this point.

Paralleling the road, this bike path measures 6-8 feet wide and has a surface of stone dust for much of the way. It starts with a mostly downhill course along the park boundary and the back yards of several homes, then widens at the 0.6-mile mark where it merges with an old road and continues past a few fields. The path narrows on a short detour around maintenance buildings at the **ranger station** and ends in an area of lawns nearby, 1.4 miles from the Gale Pond trailhead at Rte. 185.

Turn left on the pavement at the ranger station and ride uphill past the **Shadow Pond** parking and picnic area to the edge of woods, then turn right (north) on the gated road to continue the park's loop.

Cut into the side of the hill, the road climbs a steady grade for a half-mile to **Lake Louise**, a small pond perched in a saddle on the ridgeline where many riders will want to pause to admire the view while they catch their breath. The pond's natural shoreline is dominated by boggy plants and is viewed from a wooden boardwalk.

Here a short side trip forks to the right. A third of a mile in length, this dead end road climbs quickly to a point beneath **the Pinnacle**, a rock outcropping with a great view. It ends in a loop at a small clearing where a western vista is

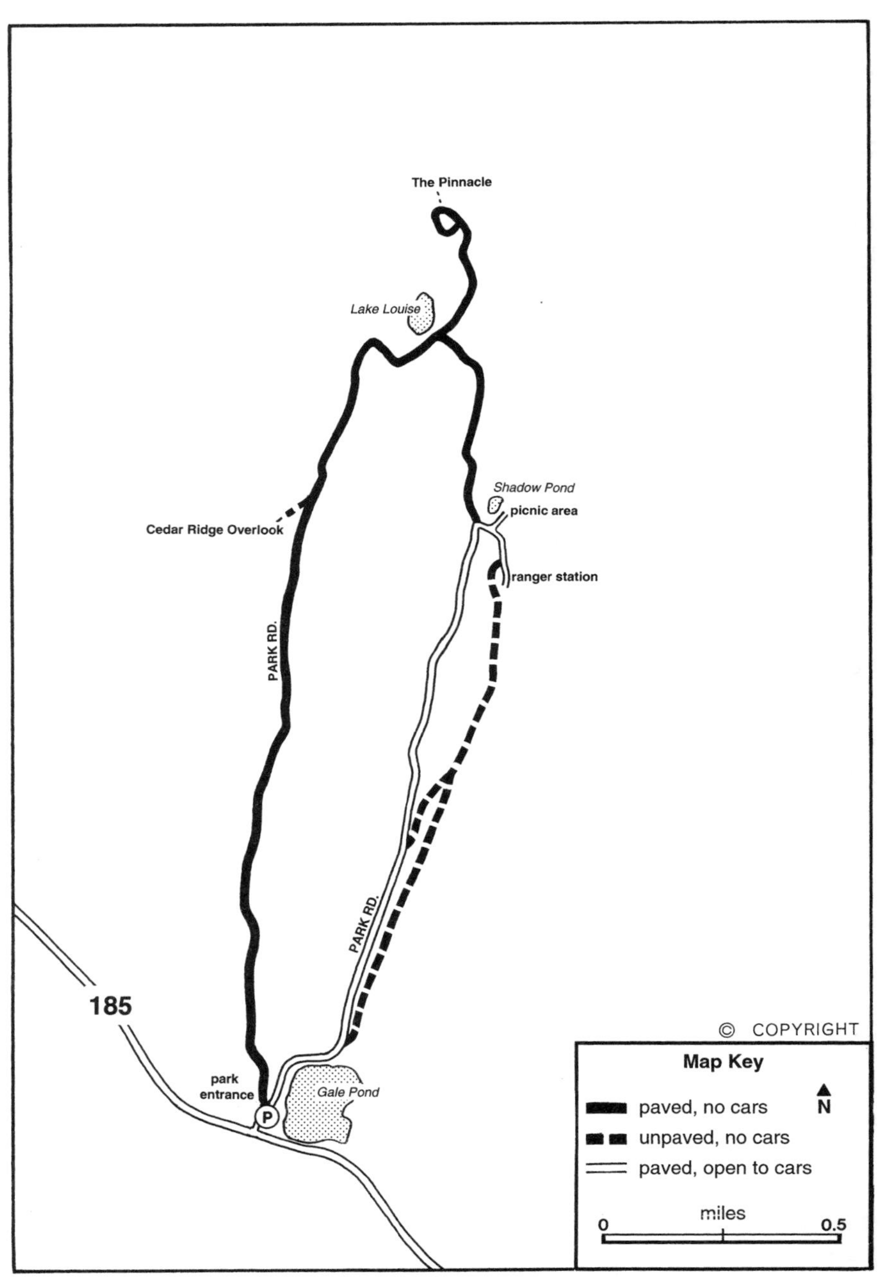

The Pinnacle
Lake Louise
Shadow Pond
picnic area
Cedar Ridge Overlook
ranger station
PARK RD.
PARK RD.
185
park
entrance
P
Gale Pond
© COPYRIGHT
Map Key
paved, no cars
unpaved, no cars
paved, open to cars
N
miles
0
0.5

visible through nearby trees, but a short hike up the blue-blazed footpath yields a better view.

Returning to the main loop, the road continues over flat ground in a westerly direction for a short distance, then turns south and begins to ascend a long slope with a crumbling surface of pavement. The road climbs for 0.4 miles, then tops the hill at a turnout for the **Cedar Ridge Overlook** where a short, unpaved side trail on the right leads uphill to a broad view of the western horizon. Use appropriate caution when visiting this open cliff face.

Continuing southward for the remaining 1.3 miles, the road descends for most of the next half-mile as it curves through the forest and passes numerous outcroppings of ledge. The pavement has deteriorated along this distance and has been replaced with a gravelly surface in places so cyclists are reminded to keep to a safe speed, especially in fall when leaves obscure the bumps. After a brief uphill, the road levels and then tips downward for most of the last half-mile to the parking lot at Gale Pond.

BACKGROUND:

Curtis H Veeder gifted this land to the state in 1944 with the hope that others could enjoy its beauty as he did. The 787-acre tract had been his summer estate and was named *Penwood* for the fact that Mr. Veeder had family roots in Pennsylvania and because the name Veeder is Dutch for *pen*.

Veeder was both a successful industrialist and an avid outdoorsman and these interests spurred him to engineer and build many of the woodland trails and roads that park visitors enjoy today. Mowed lawns and a picnic area occupy his former homesite.

DRIVING DIRECTIONS:

From I-84 take Exit 50 and follow Rte. 44 west for 2.5 miles. Turn right on Rte. 189 north and drive for 0.8 miles, then turn left on Rte. 185 west and continue for 5 miles. Look for the park entrance on the right.

TOILETS:

at Shadow Pond

ADDITIONAL INFORMATION:

Penwood State Park, 57 Gun Mill Rd., Bloomfield, CT 06002, (860) 242-1158, www.dep.state.ct.us

24 Charter Oak Landing, Great River Park

Hartford & East Hartford, CT

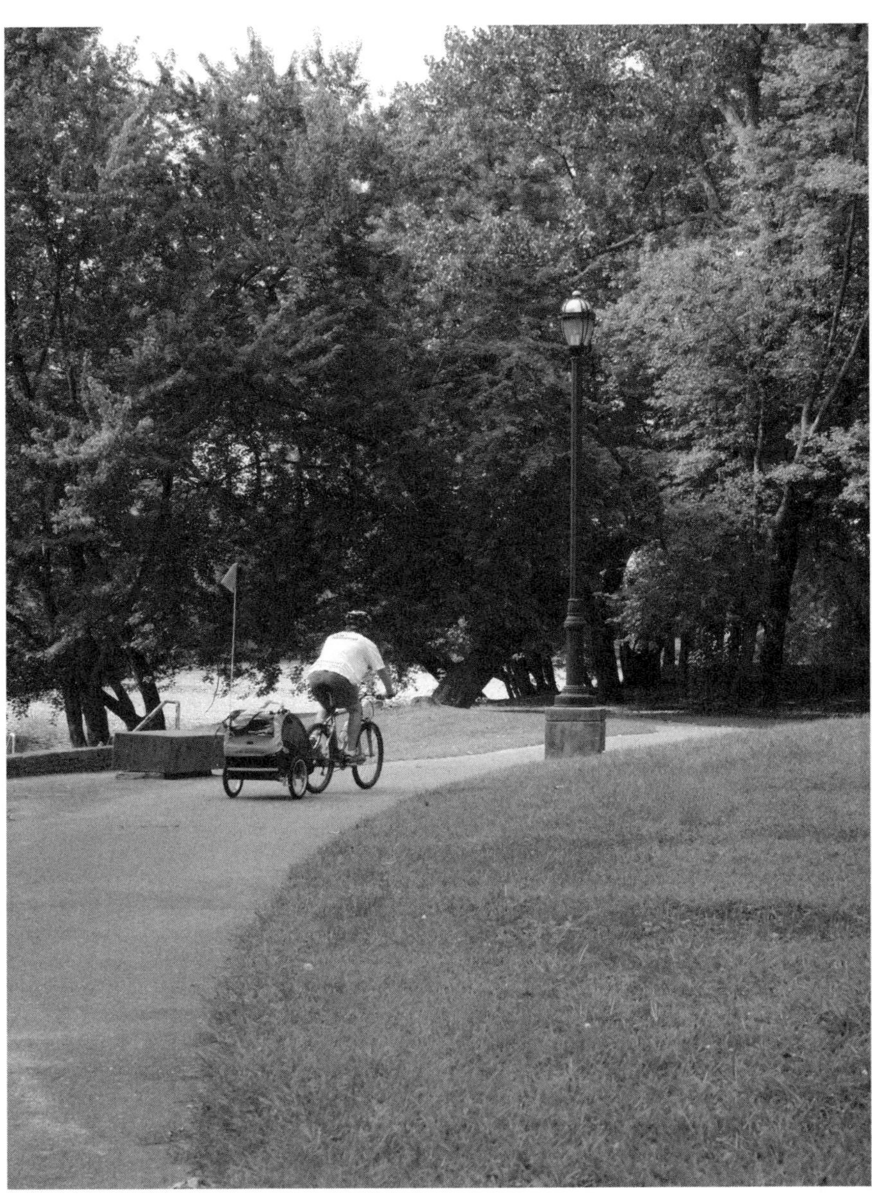

LENGTH: 4.5 miles
SURFACE: mostly pavement
TERRAIN: flat, with stairways at bridges

Green space at Hartford's front steps, these parks have transformed the banks of the Connecticut River and brought recreation to the heart of the city.

RULES & SAFETY:

- Bicyclists should yield to pedestrians.
- Keep to the right, pass on the left, and alert others (*"On your left..."*) when approaching from behind.
- Ride at a safe speed, and use extra caution in crowded areas and when children or pets are present, since their movements can be unpredictable.
- Dogs must be leashed and their wastes removed.
- Some of the trails are vulnerable to flooding during times of high water.
- The area is open during daylight hours.

ORIENTATION:

The Connecticut River is a unifying landmark which is visible from all parts of the paved trail network and divides the trails on the west bank (Hartford) from those on the east bank (East Hartford). Crossing the river is possible on the bike/pedestrian pathways of three highway bridges but involves climbing and descending long stairways, so most bicyclists choose to explore either one side or the other.

The pathway on the west side is not yet completely developed and encounters an unpaved midsection which involves a steep banking. Many points along the trails are subject to flooding during wet periods so plan your visit accordingly.

TRAIL DESCRIPTION:

The longest stretch of contiguous bike path lies on the east bank at **Great River Park**. Landscaped grounds lend a relaxing atmosphere to the park and its riverbank location provides a view of the Hartford skyline.

Heading north from the parking lot near the boat

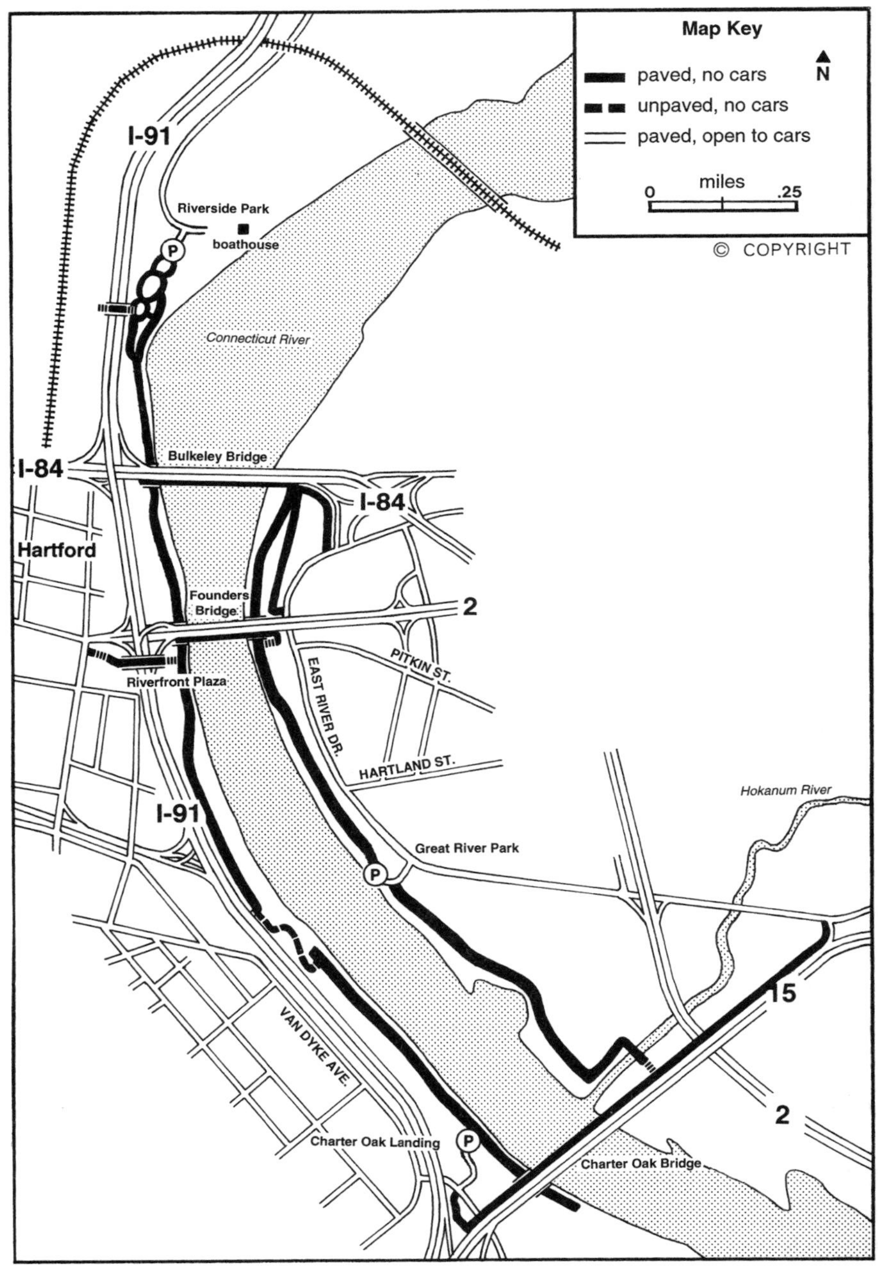
Map Key
paved, no cars
unpaved, no cars
paved, open to cars
N
miles
0
.25
© COPYRIGHT
I-91
Riverside Park
boathouse
P
Connecticut River
I-84
Bulkeley Bridge
I-84
Hartford
Founders
Bridge
2
Riverfront Plaza
EAST RIVER DR.
PITKIN ST.
HARTLAND ST.
I-91
Hokanum River
Great River Park
P
15
VAN DYKE AVE.
2
Charter Oak Landing
P
Charter Oak Bridge

ramp, the paved trail runs for 0.7 miles. It begins along a row of lamp poles in a green space corridor bound by the **Connecticut River** on one side and a 30' earthen floodwall which protects the surrounding neighborhood from flooding on the other. After a third of a mile, the trail arcs around the base of an apartment building and then passes underneath **Founders Bridge** and **Rte. 2**, where a stairway climbs to a bike and pedestrian pathway leading across the river.

Continuing northward, the trail follows more lamp poles to an area of benches overlooking the water and then veers uphill on a gradual slope to the **Bulkeley Bridge** and the roar of **I-84**. Here two short side trails branch to **East River Dr.**, one heading south along the top of the floodwall and the other running east along the Exit 53 off-ramp.

Heading south from the Great River Park parking lot, the trail offers three quarters of a mile of quieter scenery. Removed from the sights and sounds of nearby civilization, the smooth pathway meanders beside a natural border of woods lined with more lamp poles and a few benches overlooking the river.

The trail turns upstream beside the **Hokanum River** near the end, crosses its flow on a small bridge, and ends at a stairway leading to the **Charter Oak Bridge** and **Rte. 15**. At the top of the stairs, a mile of separated bike and pedestrian pathway extends along the edge of the highway from East River Dr. in East Hartford across the river to **Reserve Rd.** in Hartford, offering a view of the city and its waterfront along the way.

This pathway ends across from the entrance drive to **Charter Oak Landing** which occupies the western shoreline with lawns, picnic tables, toilets, a playground, parking lot, and a half-mile of paved pathway along the river. At the northern end of the landscaped area, a rougher foot trail continues upstream to link more paved pathways. To find it, fork left on a dirt road along the embankment below **I-91**, take the next left and climb a short, eroded slope, then turn right at the top to reach a paved access road which is closed to regular traffic.

Heading straight on this pavement, cyclists top a small hill with a view of the river and then drop to the water's edge at Hartford's **Riverfront Plaza** about 1.2 miles north of the Charter Oak Bridge. Here a pedestrian overpass spans I-91 to connect the city streets with a boat landing and outdoor performance space beside the river.

More parkland and pathway spread northward from this point. Passing under the **Founders Bridge** and **Rte. 2**, the paved trail winds through a small area of lawn, plantings, and benches for a quarter-mile then dips under the **Bulkeley Bridge** and **I-84** at a low point which is subject to flooding. When passing under this bridge, notice the high water marks placed on the abutment above the trail. A metal railing protects this section along the water.

The pathway continues through trees for another quarter-mile to a small network of paved trails at **Riverside Park**, 1.9 miles north of the Charter Oak Bridge. The park's shady grounds, picnic area, and playground make an inviting place to stop and rest.

BACKGROUND:

Hartford's waterfront had suffered during the city's growth. The arrival of the railroad in 1835 separated the riverbank from the city, the construction of a floodwall in 1942 blocked the water from view, and the completion of I-91 in 1962 added an impenetrable barrier.

The "Riverfront Recapture" effort to reclaim public access and restore the city's connection to the river started in 1981 and continues today. The first portions of the so-called riverwalk system were achieved when the city of Hartford completed Charter Oak Landing in 1989 and East Hartford opened Great River Park in 1990. The initiative reached a major milestone in 1999 when Riverfront Plaza, Founders Bridge Promenade, and State St. Landing were dedicated. In the shadow of the city skyline, paved trails, outdoor performance areas, boat landings, and picnic areas now invite people to enjoy the river and its banks.

The Metropolitan District Commission (MDC) and Riverfront Recapture, Inc. manage and maintain the area.

DRIVING DIRECTIONS:

Great River Park from I-84 westbound: Take Exit 54 and follow Rte. 2 west toward downtown Hartford. Take Exit 3, turn left at the end of the ramp on Darlin St., then turn left on East River Dr. The parking lot is 0.8 miles ahead on the right.

Great River Park from I-84 eastbound: Take Exit 53 and follow signs for East River Dr. Turn right off the ramp and continue on East River Dr. for 0.7 miles to the parking lot on the right.

Charter Oak Landing from I-91 northbound: Take Exit 27 and turn left (north) on Brainard Rd. After 0.8 miles, turn left on Reserve Rd. and continue for a half-mile to the park entrance on the right.

Charter Oak Landing from i-91 southbound: Take Exit 27 and turn left off the ramp on Airport Rd. Turn left on Brainard Rd. and drive for 0.7 miles, then left on Reserve Rd. and continue for a half-mile to the park entrance on the right.

Riverside Park from I-91: Take Exit 33 and turn east on Jennings Rd. Turn right (south) on Leibert Rd. and look for the park entrance 0.4 miles ahead on the left.

TOILETS:

Great River Park, Charter Oak Landing, Riverside Park

ADDITIONAL INFORMATION:

Metropolitan District Commission (MDC), P.O. Box 800, Hartford, CT 06142-0800, (860) 278-7850, www.themdc.com

Riverfront Recapture, Inc., (860) 713-3131, www.riverfront.org

25 Windsor Center River Trail

Windsor, CT

LENGTH: 1.4 miles
SURFACE: paved
TERRAIN: flat

Curving through trees on the banks of the Farmington River, this loop is well suited for a ride with small kids. A few low-lying points are vulnerable to river flooding.

RULES & SAFETY:

- Bicyclists should yield to pedestrians.
- Keep to the right, pass on the left, and ride at a safe speed. Remember that the loop has two-way traffic.
- Be extra careful in the presence of children and pets since their movements can be unpredictable.
- Alert others *("On your left...")* when approaching from behind to avoid startling them.
- Pets must be leashed and their wastes removed.
- The area is open only during daylight hours.

ORIENTATION:

Crossing no roads, the trail forms a mile-long loop with two spurs. Trail intersections have signs pointing to the destinations displayed on the accompanying map.

TRAIL DESCRIPTION:

Start from the trailhead on **Palisado Ave.** (**Rte. 159**). Following the loop in the clockwise direction (forking left), the trail curves through woods on a faint downslope, reaching a T-intersection beside the **Farmington River** after 0.2 miles.

To the left (north), a spur trail runs for a quarter-mile to **Pleasant St. Park**, crossing a bridge over **Mill Brook**, losing its paved surface, and passing under Rte. 159 along the way. To the right (south), the main loop follows the river downstream in the shade of tall trees, then turns west and emerges at an arched bridge and a second T-intersection.

Here another spur heads left to connect **Mechanic St.**

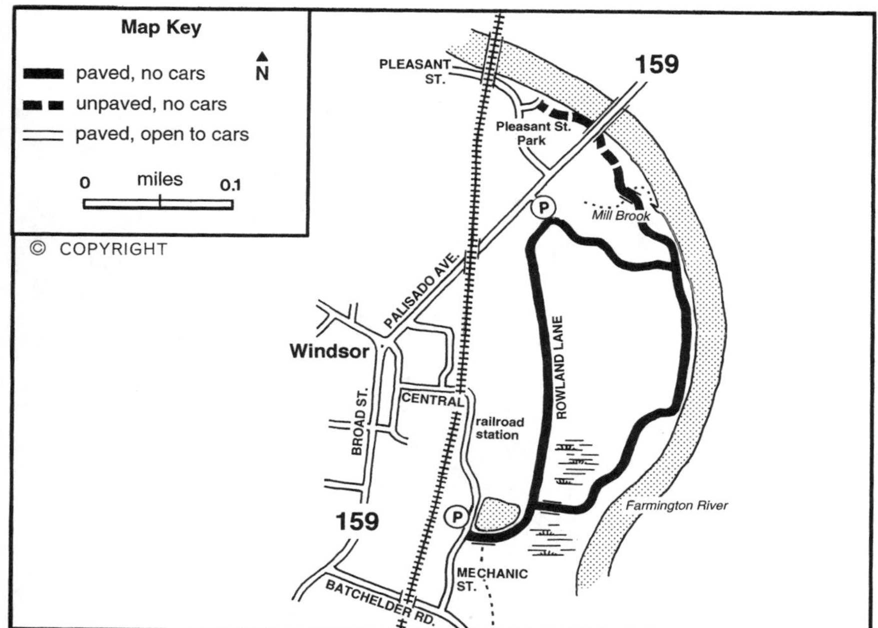

near a public parking lot and the downtown business area, while the main loop returns to the right (north) on 0.4-mile stretch of a colonial era road bed known as **Rowland Lane**.

BACKGROUND:

The town of Windsor began creating this trail in 1993 with its engineering department managing the project, and opened the trail for public use in 1996. The trail utilizes a 43-acre town-owned parcel of land and includes Rowland Lane, an abandoned public road dating from colonial times which had once been the main route along the Connecticut River from Hartford to points north.

DRIVING DIRECTIONS:

From I-91 take Exit 38 and follow Rte. 75 south for 2 miles to Windsor Center. Turn left (north) at the traffic signal on Rte. 159 north and drive for a quarter-mile to the parking lot on the right, just before a bridge over the Farmington River.

TOILETS:

none on-site

ADDITIONAL INFORMATION:

Windsor Town Hall, (860) 285-1800

26 Windsor Locks Canal State Park

Suffield - Windsor Locks, CT

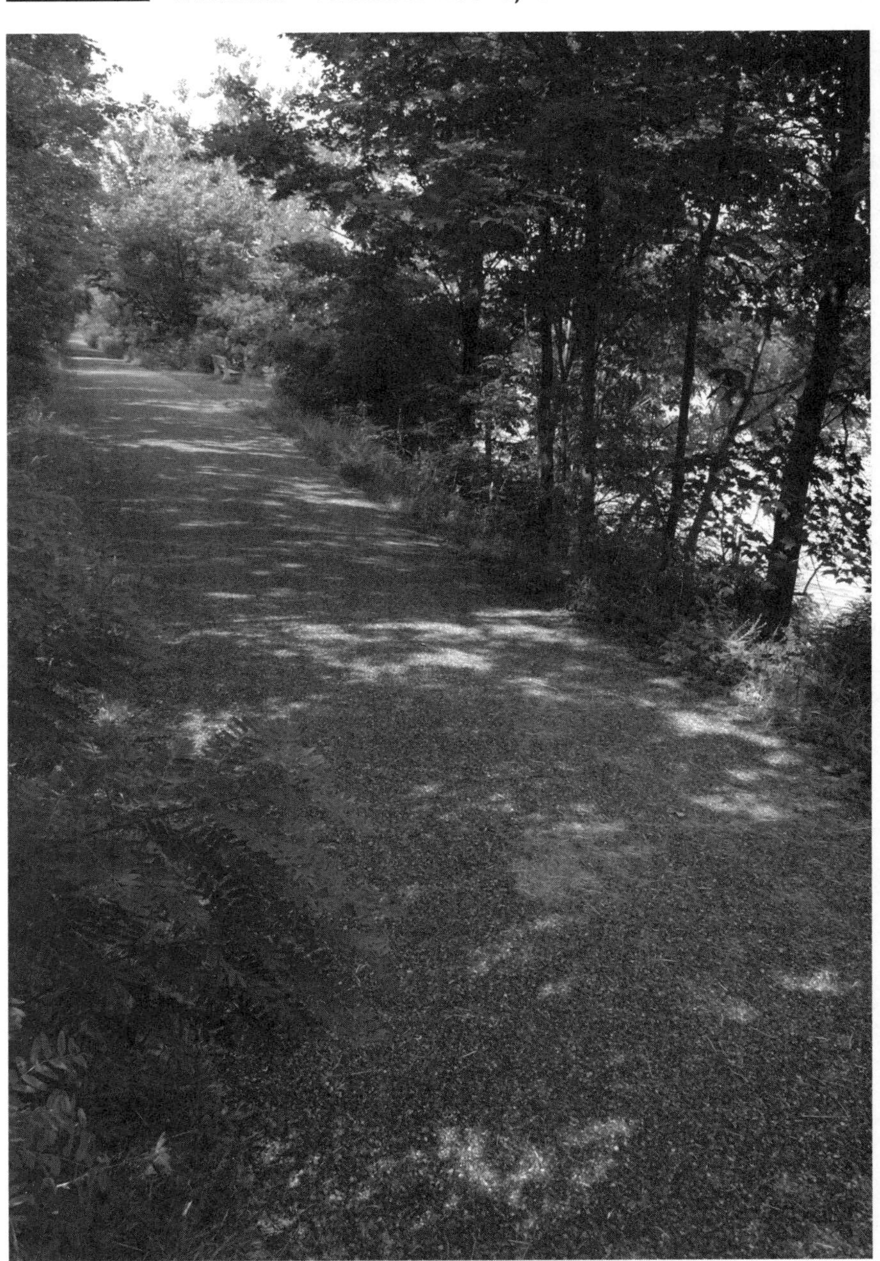

LENGTH: 5.5 miles
SURFACE: paved
TERRAIN: mostly flat
NOTE: closed annually from mid-November until early April

Combining natural scenery with an interesting relic of history, the Windsor Locks Canal Towpath delivers an easy ride along the Connecticut River. A new adjoining bike path extends the riding across the river to Enfield.

RULES & SAFETY:

• The towpath is closed from mid-November until early April each year in order to protect endangered birds of prey. Chainlink gates are locked at each endpoint during this time to prevent entry.

• Signs warn visitors to *"Pass at your own risk."*

• The trail is relatively isolated. Since water confines both sides, it is accessible only at the two ends and cannot be entered or exited from any point in between.

• Be aware that steep, unprotected bankings are a potential hazard beside the trail in several places, especially for small children.

• Alert others (*"On your left..."*) when approaching from behind to avoid startling them.

• The park is open only during daylight hours.

ORIENTATION:

Both the 4.4-mile Windsor Locks Canal Towpath and the adjoining 1.1-mile Enfield-Suffield Bike Path intersect no roads, but otherwise they differ noticeably. The towpath enjoys the state park's flat, peaceful, and natural scenery along the canal but dense growth along its route allows surprisingly few views of the river. The hillier Enfield-Suffield Bike Path follows the edge of a busy roadway and crosses a bridge over the river for an unbroken view.

Mileage marks painted on the towpath's pavement at half-mile increments originate at the northern terminus, the most popular trailhead. Additional parking is available at the towpath's southern terminus off Rte. 140.

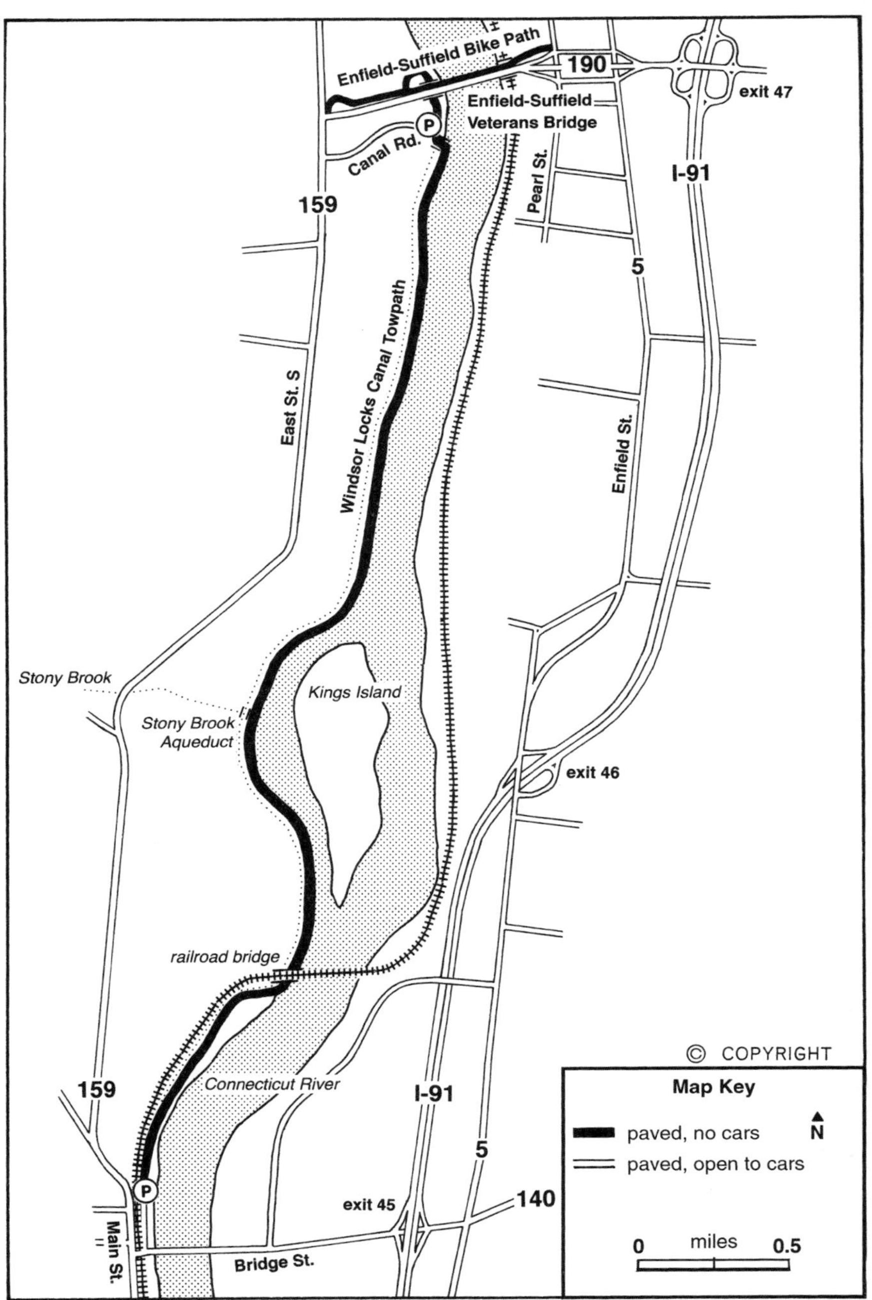

Enfield-Suffield Bike Path
190
exit 47
Enfield-Suffield
Veterans Bridge
Canal Rd.
P
Pearl St.
I-91
159
5
Windsor Locks Canal Towpath
East St. S
Enfield St.
Stony Brook
Kings Island
Stony Brook
Aqueduct
exit 46
railroad bridge
© COPYRIGHT
Map Key
paved, no cars
N
paved, open to cars
159
Connecticut River
I-91
5
P
140
exit 45
Main St.
Bridge St.
0
miles
0.5

TRAIL DESCRIPTION:

Beginning at the **Canal Rd.** trailhead in Suffield, turn south (right, when facing the river) to follow the **Windsor Locks Canal Towpath**. The trail first crosses a bridge over the start of the canal with an upstream view of the **Connecticut River**, the rapids known as Enfield Falls, and the head of the canal. Painted mileage markers originate from this point.

The pathway travels along the crest of a banking created when the canal was dug and follows a fairly straight line beside the river for the first 1.8 miles. Water in the canal borders the right side of the trail and the broad flow of the Connecticut is visible through trees on the left. Note that a steep banking drops from the trail's pavement to the river's edge and deserves appropriate caution since no protective fencing exists for trail users.

Less than a mile from the trailhead, notice that the terrain beside the trail steepens and the canal hugs the base of a high slope. Carved from the hillside in a massive effort, the canal's even, level channel is easily appreciated while rolling along this section of the towpath.

The trail arcs to the right after 1.8 miles where the river splits at **Kings Island** and it continues for the next 1.3 miles beside a narrower stretch of water which flows past the west side of the island.

Look for the **Stony Brook Aqueduct** ahead at the 2.3-mile mark. One of the canal's most impressive features, the aqueduct forms a bridge for the water in the canal to pass six feet over the flow of **Stony Brook**, a tributary stream which crosses perpendicularly. The aqueduct consists of huge stone supports and a bed of wooden beams which have recently been reinforced with a layer of concrete. The towpath crosses the brook a few feet away on a parallel bridge.

The trail leaves the shore of the river at this point for the next half-mile, then returns to the edge of another steep banking above the water and continues past the southern tip of Kings Island. Glimpses across the full width of the river appear through gaps in the trees.

At the 3.3-mile mark, the towpath enters Windsor Locks as it passes underneath a **railroad bridge** which spans both the canal and the river and serves an active rail line carrying both passenger and freight trains. Here the trail leaves the edge of the river again, turns hard right at a stone bridge abutment, and heads westward with the canal along the contours of the land.

The last mile of trail turns back to the south and returns to the sights and sounds of civilization. The river, towpath, canal, and railroad run shoulder-to-shoulder along the final stretch with a wall of dense brush blocking most views. The trail ends at a gate and parking lot beside a mill complex off **Rte. 140**.

North of the canal, the adjoining **Enfield-Suffield Bike Path** connects communities on both sides of the river with the state park. Heading north (left, when facing the river) from the Canal Rd. trailhead parking lot, it dips under a bridge for **Rte. 190** and reverses direction in a broad turn which climbs to the side of the roadway and splits at the quarter-mile mark. Turning left (east), the path follows the edge of Rte. 190 across the **Enfield-Suffield Veterans Bridge** to reach **Pearl St.** in Enfield after a half-mile. Turning right (west), it runs for a third of a mile to **Rte. 159** in Suffield.

BACKGROUND:

The Windsor Locks Canal was built by hand between 1827 and 1829. Over 400 Irish immigrants dug the 5.5-mile channel using shovels and wheel barrows, excavating dirt and rock along a slope beside the river and piling it to form the banking that would become the towpath.

The canal's depth was four and a half feet and its width was 80 feet, wide enough to accommodate steamboats. Three locks were built to bridge the 30-foot elevation change in the river and an aqueduct, still functioning, carries the canal above Stony Brook, a tributary stream. Originally, horses and mules pulled the boat traffic along the canal using the towpath.

The canal enabled boats to avoid Enfield Falls, a series of rapids which had marked the northernmost point on the river navigable by sea-going vessels. Its creation enhanced trade between the sea-coast and inland areas including Vermont and Canada and served local industry until 1845, when the railroad arrived. It then continued functioning as a power source for nearby mills.

Today, portions of the canal and towpath are owned and managed cooperatively by Northeast Utilities, the state of Connecticut, the Nature Conservancy, and the Dexter Corporation.

The Enfield-Suffield bike path was added in 2010 in conjunction with road and bridge construction. The town of Enfield has proposed a future extension of the trail on the east side of the river.

DRIVING DIRECTIONS:

From I-91 take Exit 47W. Follow Rte. 190 west for 1.3 miles, then turn left on Rte. 159 south. Take the next left on Canal St. and park in the lot at the end.

TOILETS:

portable toilet (seasonal) at the Canal St. trailhead.

ADDITIONAL INFORMATION:

Connecticut Dept. of Environmental Protection, (860) 424-3200, www.ct.gov/dep

27 Capt. John Bissell Greenway

East Hartford - Windsor, CT

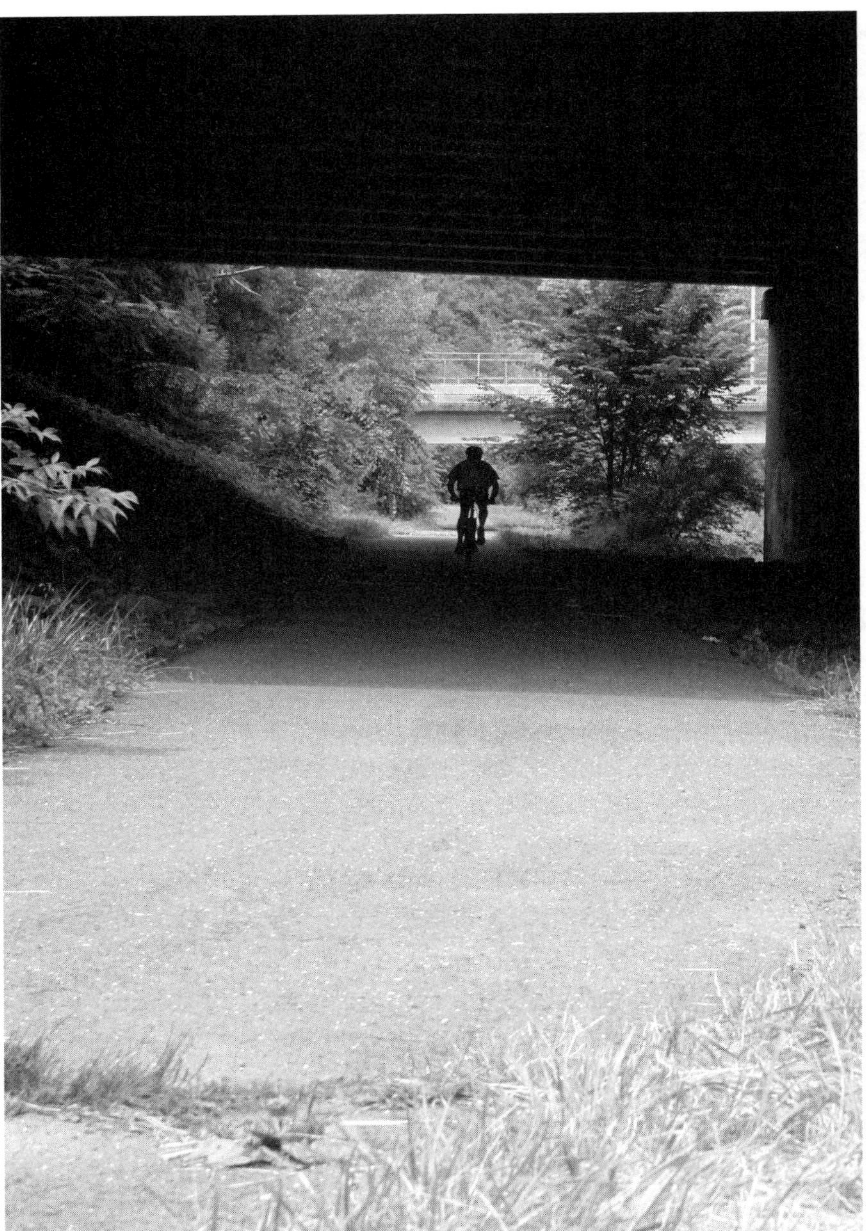

LENGTH: 7.4 miles (includes 2.9-mile on-road segment)
SURFACE: paved
TERRAIN: moderate hills

In heroic style, the Capt. John Bissell Greenway dodges the ramps and overpasses of 3 interstate highways and spans the Connecticut River with a safe passageway for self-propelled travelers. If you don't mind the highway noise, an on-road segment, and a few hills, it's easy to appreciate what this path delivers.

RULES & SAFETY:

• Hills and limited visibility at corners make it important to ride at a safe speed and to remember that the bike path has two-way traffic.

• Keep to the right, pass on the left, and alert others (*"On your left..."*) when approaching from behind to avoid startling them.

• When crossing roads, stop before entering the roadway and assume that drivers do not see you.

• Help keep it clean: carry out all that you carry in.

ORIENTATION:

The Capt. John Bissell Greenway spans the 7.4-mile distance from the Charter Oak Greenway (Chapter 28) in East Hartford at the southeast end to Windsor Meadows State Park in Windsor at the northwest end. Much of this route involves a separated pathway but a 2.9-mile segment along the midsection is only a marked, on-road bike route. The southeastern section of separated bike path measures 3.1 miles long and holds the hilliest, curviest conditions as well as the greatest visual separation from surrounding highways. The northwestern end of the bike path measures 1.4 miles long and follows the side of a highway as it crosses the Connecticut River.

Wickham Park (seasonal) is a good starting point for the greenway. A small entrance fee is charged and the park is open daily from 9:30 AM until dusk from early April through late October. At the greenway's northwestern end, Windsor

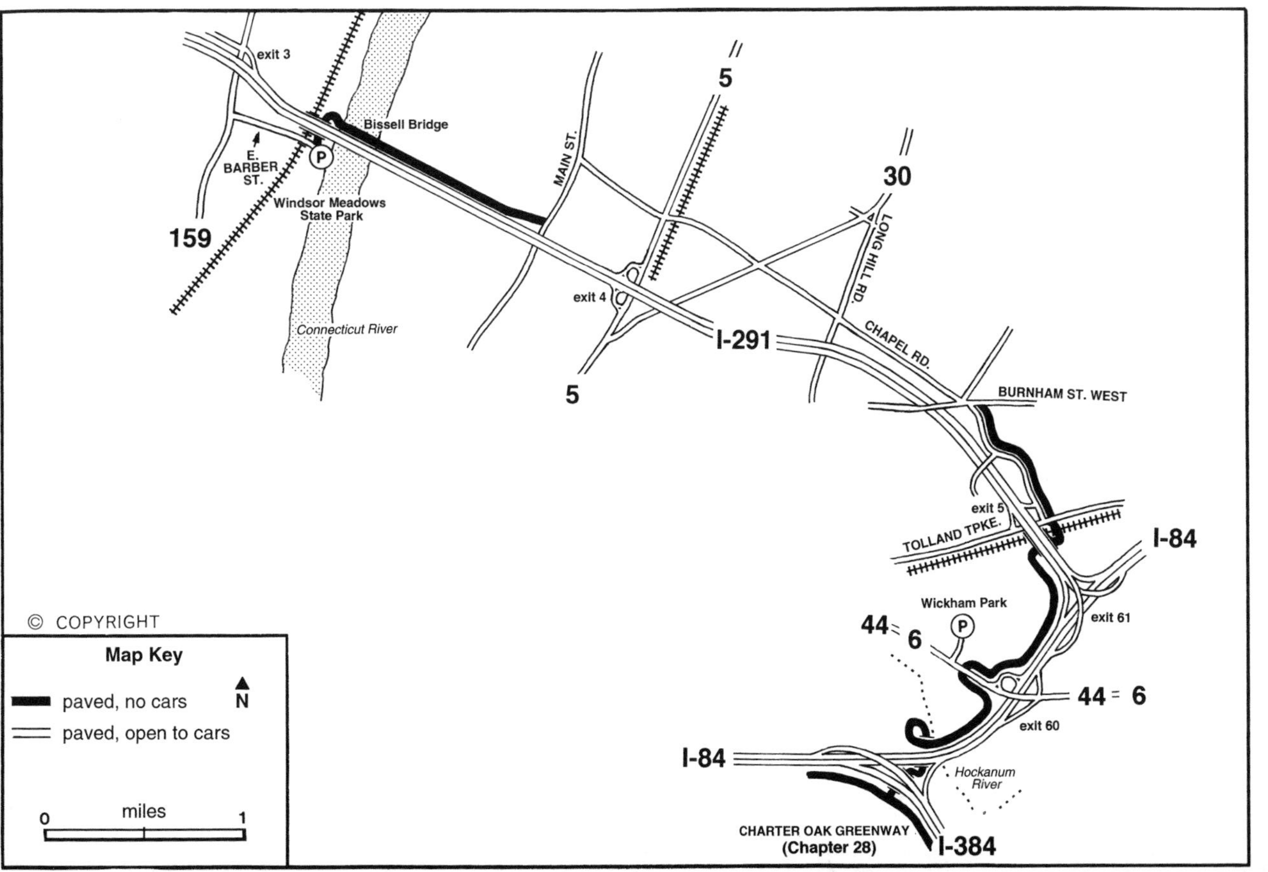

exit 3
E. BARBER ST.
159
Windsor Meadows State Park
Bissell Bridge
Connecticut River
MAIN ST.
exit 4
5
5
I-291
30
LONG HILL RD.
CHAPEL RD.
BURNHAM ST. WEST
exit 5
TOLLAND TPKE.
Wickham Park
44 6
I-84
exit 61
44 6
exit 60
Hockanum River
I-384
CHARTER OAK GREENWAY
(Chapter 28)
I-84
© COPYRIGHT
Map Key
paved, no cars
paved, open to cars
N
0
miles
1

Meadows State Park serves as an alternate trailhead.

The bike path varies between 10 and 14 feet wide, has an aging paved surface, and is bordered by protective fencing where necessary. Signs point to destinations at points along the way and crosswalks exist where the bike path meets roads. The on-road midsection of the greenway is clearly marked by green *Bike Route* signs posted at intersections.

TRAIL DESCRIPTION:

Begin in Manchester at **Wickham Park**, a 250-acre property which was once the home of Clarence H. Wickham, a local industrialist who desired that it become a parkland for all to enjoy. Managed by a private organization, the park offers picnic areas, manicured grounds, fields, gardens, and an excellent view over the Hartford area.

Leaving the Wickham Park entrance gate, turn left beside **Rte. 44** to reach the bike path. To follow it in the southeast direction, cross Rte. 44 and continue along the path as it parallels the roadway then veers to the right near a highway off-ramp. It follows the broad turns of this roadway for most of the first half-mile with earthen embankments and foliage buffering the trail from the sight of traffic for most of the way.

Descending, it eventually merges with the edge of the roadway, crosses a bridge over the **Hockanum River**, and then turns 270 degrees in a loop which redirects the path under the highway bridge beside the river. Climbing a strenuous slope into East Hartford on the other side, the path joins a barrier at the edge of **I-84** for a short distance and then turns south, passes under a ramp for **I-384**, and ends after 1.1 miles at the **Charter Oak Greenway** (Chapter 28).

Heading in the opposite direction from Wickham Park, the trail follows a wooden fence beside Rte. 44 for a tenth of a mile, then turns left and begins a half-mile climb which starts beside a highway off-ramp and later enters its own space bound by earthen bankings on both sides. After topping this hill, the path descends for a short distance to the side of **I-291** where protective fencing leads it over mostly flat ground.

Near the 1-mile mark, the path turns and passes underneath a bridge carrying the highway over a set of railroad tracks and the **Tolland Tpke.**, then crosses the tracks and the turnpike at a crosswalk and continues beside **Chapel Rd.** in an industrial park. The paved surface of the bike path is badly cracked along this portion. After following Chapel Rd. for about a mile, the path ends near the intersection of **Burnham St.**, 2 miles from Wickham Park.

A marked, on-road bike route continues into South Windsor from this point for the next 2.9 miles. It follows Chapel Rd. for 2.5 miles to the end, then turns left (south) on **Main St.** for another 0.4 miles. Although the route crosses a few busy roads, it holds moderate traffic levels and remains in mostly residential areas. Green *Bike Route* signs bearing the image of a bicycle mark the way.

Look for the separated bike path resuming on the right side just before Main St. passes underneath a bridge for I-291. The path ascends gradually beside a metal fence to the side of the highway and follows it closely for the remaining 1.4 miles. Protected by fencing and barriers, bicyclists pedal safely alongside the traffic and eventually cross the **Connecticut River** on the **Capt. John Bissell Bridge** where views of New England's largest river and the Hartford skyline await.

Reaching the west side of the river, the trail turns and descends beneath the highway at another set of railroad tracks and soon ends at **Windsor Meadows State Park**, 6.3 miles from Wickham Park. Windsor Meadows is a popular boat launching site and serves as an alternate trailhead for the bike path.

BACKGROUND:

The greenway is named for Capt. John Bissell (1591-1677), founder of Windsor, CT. It was created in 1996 in conjunction with the construction of I-291 in an effort to improve bicycle and pedestrian transportation in the area.

Although the trail is free of the high traffic levels found at some of the region's other bike paths, it will undoubtedly become busier as greater Hartford's network of bike and pedestrian routes expands. Future construction at the greenway's northwest endpoint will create a trail running south along the river from Windsor Meadows State Park to Riverside Park in Hartford (Chapter 24). And at the opposite end, extensions to the Charter Oak Greenway are expected to link East Hartford's Great River Park (Chapter 24) with the Hop River State Park Tr. (Chapter 30).

DRIVING DIRECTIONS:

- **Wickham Park (seasonal) from I-84:** Take Exit 60 and follow Rte. 44 west. Look for the park entrance immediately ahead on the right.
- **Windsor Meadows from I-291 westbound:** Take Exit 3 and follow signs to Rte. 159 south. After a third of a mile on Rte. 159 south, turn left on E. Barber St. and park at the end.
- **Windsor Meadows from I-91 northbound:** Take Exit 34 and follow signs to Rte. 159. Turn right on Rte. 159 north and drive for 0.7 miles, then turn right on E. Barber St. and continue to the end.
- **Windsor Meadows from I-91 southbound:** Take Exit 35B and follow Rte. 218 east for a half-mile. Turn right on Rte. 159 south and drive for a third of a mile, then turn left on E. Barber St. and continue to the end.

TOILETS:

in season at Wickham Park and Windsor Meadows State Park

ADDITIONAL INFORMATION:

Wickham Park, 1329 West Middle Tpke., Manchester, CT 06040, (860) 528-0856, www.wickhampark.org

Connecticut Dept. of Environmental Protection, www.ct.gov/dep

28 Charter Oak Greenway

East Hartford - Manchester, CT

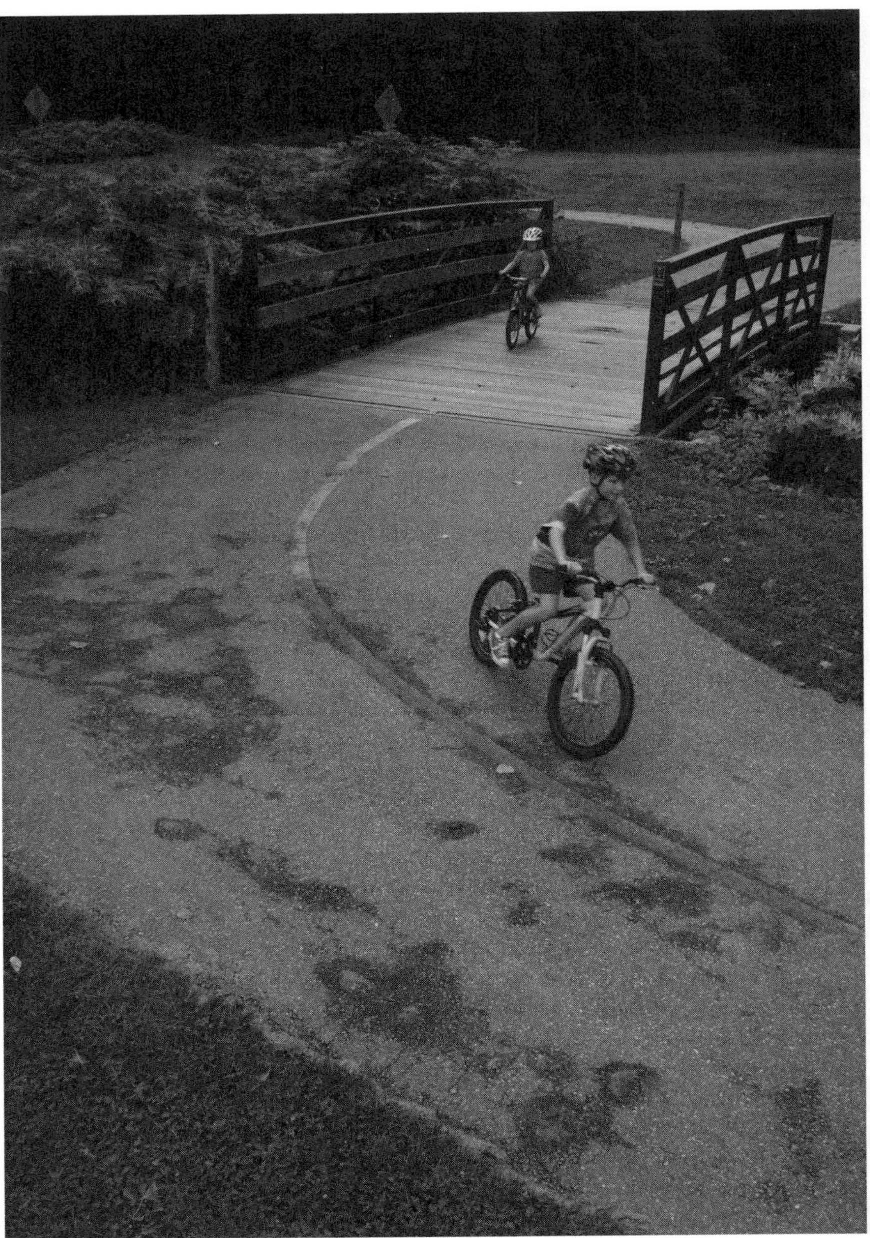

LENGTH: 7.5 miles (including on-road segments)
SURFACE: paved
TERRAIN: hilly

This rolling ribbon of asphalt allows great connections as it weaves through parks, highway interchanges, and a variety of places in between. Traffic noise and short on-road segments are occasional disruptions.

RULES & SAFETY:

• Bicyclists should yield to pedestrians.

• The bike path is narrow in places and encounters steep slopes and blind corners. Keep to the right side, ride at a safe speed, and always be ready to encounter others.

• Be especially cautious in the presence of children and pets since their movements can be unpredictable.

• Alert others (*"On your left..."*) when approaching from behind to avoid startling them.

• Step off the trail when stopped so that others can pass unimpeded.

• Respect the private property along the trail.

• Stop at road intersections and assume that drivers do not see you.

• Dogs must be leashed and their wastes removed.

ORIENTATION:

The Charter Oak Greenway is an east-west route from Forbes St. in East Hartford (western terminus) to Highland St. in Manchester (eastern terminus) utilizing a combination of separated pathways and 3 short, on-road bike routes. Paralleling I-84 and I-384 for most of this distance, the greenway encounters hills, curves, and intersections as it mingles with bridges, highway exit ramps, and surrounding properties. Numerous side trails branch along the way to connect nearby parks and neighborhoods. Bring a map when visiting for the first time and keep track of your location as you ride.

The 10'-wide trail has a border of mowed grass on each side, protective fencing where necessary, and

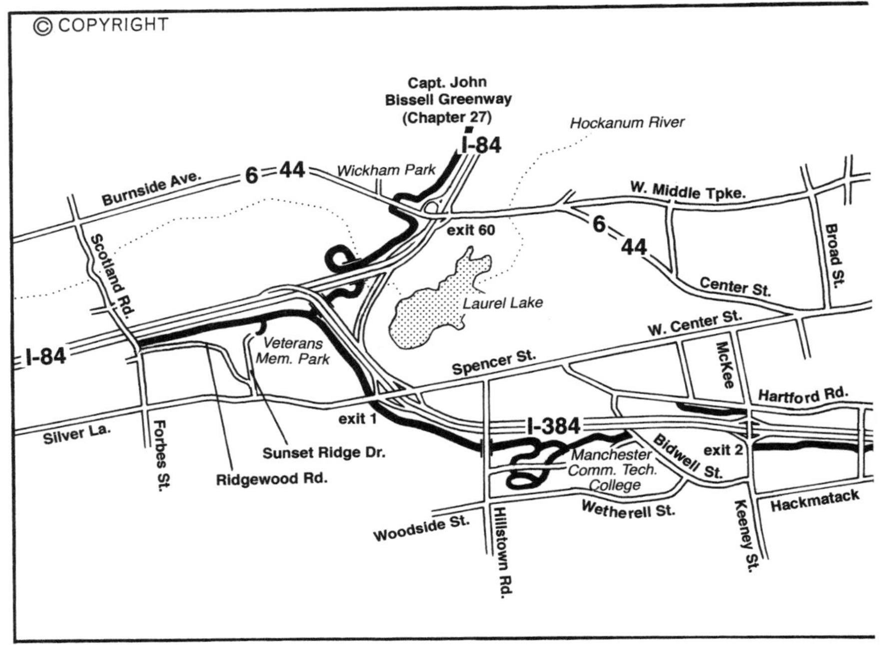

crosswalks at road intersections. On-road segments and intersections are marked by green *Bike Route* signs.

TRAIL DESCRIPTION:

Beginning at **Charter Oak Park** in Manchester, cross the playing field area from the parking lot to reach the trail. Turning east (left when facing the trail from the parking lot), the greenway extends for 1.8 miles with a mostly uphill route, much of it newly constructed. Crossing a bridge over a brook, the trail immediately forks left from a spur running uphill (south) to an **I-384** underpass and the **Mt. Nebo Playing Field**. The greenway heads east into woods on flat ground between the brook and the highway, passing a few apartment buildings before reaching a second fork at 0.6 miles where a side trail branches left to West Gardner St.

The main trail continues straight under the **Gardner St.** bridge. Crossing another bridge over the brook, it climbs two steep slopes and then curves northward for a short distance to the intersection of the highway's westbound **Exit**

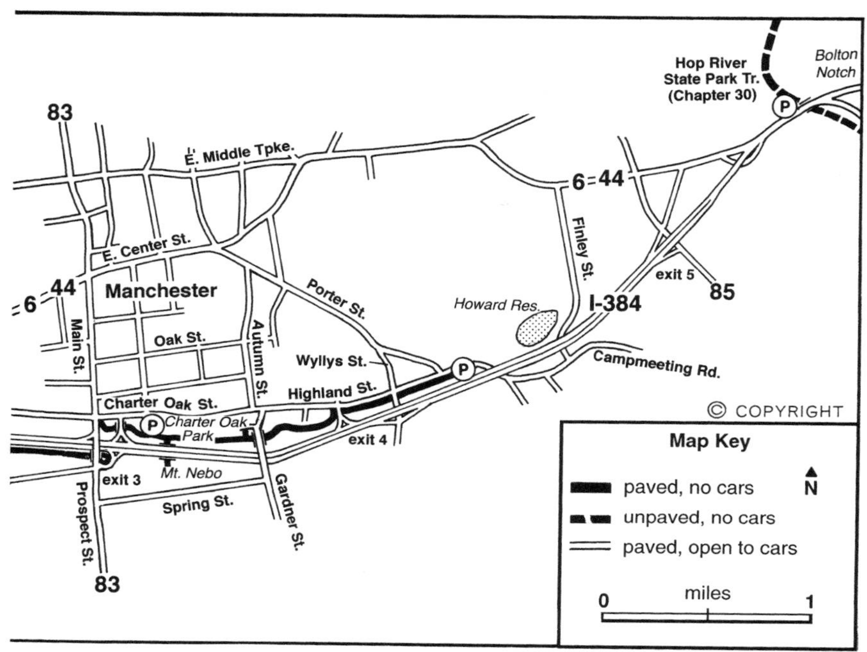

4 on/off-ramps at **Highland St.** (1.1 miles). The trail continues west on an uphill slope along a grassy strip beside the street to the intersection of **Wyllys St.** (1.5 miles) where it passes a cluster of benches and picnic tables across from a market. Much of the final third of a mile is an uphill ride to a trailhead parking lot (1.8 miles) near **Porter St.**

Heading west from Charter Oak Park (to the right when facing the trail from the parking lot), the greenway extends for 5.7 miles with greater proximity to roads and highways, including 3 short on-road sections. The trip begins along the southern edge of the park's playing fields, dipping under the highway's westbound ramps for **Exit 3** before emerging at the intersection of **Charter Oak St.** and **Main St.** (**Rte. 83**).

Turn hard left at this point and continue south along Main St. (crossing I-384) and look for a *Bike Route* sign marking the next section of the greenway on the left before the next highway off-ramp. The bike path turns on a downslope beside the exit ramp and passes underneath Main St. It follows the edge of I-384 for a third of a mile, climbs a slope to cross **Prospect St.** (1.3 miles), descends back to the side of the highway, and then rises to **Keeney St.** (1.8 miles) at the ramps for **Exit 2**.

Here a second on-road section brings the greenway back to the north side of the interstate. Following more *Bike Route* signs, turn right on Keeney and look for the bike path resuming ahead on the left before **Hartford Rd.**

The trail follows a landscaped strip of green space for a half-mile and then ends beside Hartford Rd. where the last, and longest, on-road section begins. After crossing the street, continue riding west on Hartford Rd. for a third of a mile, turn left on **Bidwell St.** (2.8 miles), cross under the highway, and find the bike path resuming on the right.

It starts with a strenuous uphill which returns riders to the side of the interstate, then turns and descends through woods to the campus of **Manchester Community Technical College**. Curving between playing fields, parking lots, and quiet woodlands on a mile-long detour from the highway, the greenway enjoys some of its most peaceful surroundings along this distance. A few intersecting paths link the campus and provide alternative loops to the main trail.

The greenway returns to the side of I-384, passes under **Hillstown Rd.** (3.9 miles), then follows a ramp for **Exit 1** to the intersection of **Silver La./Spencer St.** (4.4 miles) near the East Hartford border. After crossing, it descends in a straight line along a wooden sound barrier beside the interstate, climbs a half-mile uphill, and joins the side of **I-84**. Halfway up this slope it intersects the **Capt. John Bissell Greenway** (Chapter 27), a 7.4-mile route to Windsor.

At the top, the greenway gets a view of the Hartford skyline and intersects a side trail on the left linking **Veterans Memorial Park**, then tips downhill for the remaining distance with greater separation from the highway and wooden sound barriers blocking the noise of the traffic. It currently ends at **Forbes St.**, 5.7 miles from the Charter Oak Park trailhead.

BACKGROUND:

The Charter Oak Greenway was conceived in 1972 during the planning stages for the construction of I-384. Early visionaries promoted a safe passageway beside the highway to enable bicyclists, walkers, runners, and other human-powered travelers to reach their destinations and in 1994 it became a reality. More recently, the greenway has extended eastward from Charter Oak Park including construction of the present terminus at Highland St. in 2011.

The Charter Oak Greenway forms an important part of a growing network of bike/pedestrian pathways in the greater Hartford area. It intersects the Capt. John Bissell Greenway (Chapter 27), and is planned to be extended westward to link Great River Park in East Hartford (Chapter 24) and eastward to the Hop River State Park Tr. in Bolton (Chapter 30). It is designated as part of the East Coast Greenway, a 2600-mile route planned from Maine to Florida.

The greenway is named for one of Connecticut's most famous hiding places. In 1687 when the King's agents arrived in Hartford with armed force demanding to take the Charter from the General Court of Connecticut, daring colonials hid the document inside an old oak tree nearby. The Charter Oak no longer stands but it remains one of the state's most enduring symbols of liberty.

DRIVING DIRECTIONS:

I-384 eastbound: Take Exit 3, turn right off the ramp, and follow Main St. north to the first traffic signal. Turn right on Charter Oak St. and continue to the next traffic signal, then turn right at the entrance to Charter Oak Park.

I-384 westbound: Take Exit 3, turn right off the ramp on Charter Oak St., continue to the next traffic signal, then turn right at the entrance to Charter Oak Park.

TOILETS:

in season at Charter Oak Park

ADDITIONAL INFORMATION:

Manchester Parks & Recreation, (860) 647-3084

29 Hammonassett Beach State Park

Madison, CT

LENGTH: 2 miles
SURFACE: mostly stone dust
TERRAIN: flat

Hammonassett's main attraction is its long, ocean beach but its bike path motivates many visitors to get up and ride, walk, or run through the beautiful coastal scenery and cool sea breezes. The park's campground offers overnight possibilities.

RULES & SAFETY:

- Bicyclists should yield to pedestrians.
- Keep to the right, pass on the left, and alert others (*"On your left..."*) when approaching from behind.
- Ride at a safe speed, and use extra caution in crowded areas and when children or pets are present.
- Watch for walkers crossing the bike path at the beach access points.
- Bicyclists are requested to avoid damaging the fragile environment of the surrounding dunes and marshes. Ride only on roads and bike paths, and not on beach boardwalks.
- An entrance fee is charged during the summer season.
- The park closes at sunset each day.

ORIENTATION:

The area offers a few options for bicyclists. The most popular is the park's 1.3-mile stone dust bike path along the dunes by the beach, which is relatively exposed to sun and wind but enjoys proximity to ocean scenery and numerous comfort stations along the way. The 0.8-mile loop at Willard's Island is a quieter alternative on old paved roads which explore marshland along the Hammonassett River. A 1-mile section of the Shoreline Greenway, currently under construction with a stone dust surface, will offer a rolling, turning route through nearby woods.

TRAIL DESCRIPTION:

Begin at **West Beach**, Hammonassett's largest parking area. Facing the water, the bike path runs to the right (north) for only a tenth of a mile before ending at a picnic pavilion, but to the left (south) it extends for 1.2 miles to the end of the beach.

Following the path southward, the bike path follows sand dunes which separate it from the shoreline with a green swathe of grasses, cedars, and beach roses. A mowed field occupies the other side of the trail with picnic tables and plenty of room to play. After a third of a mile, the bike path arcs past the **Central Pavilion** where toilets and a large deck with tables are housed in a modern, concrete structure.

The trail returns to natural surroundings for most of the next 0.3 miles to the **East Beach** parking lot and beach house where a long, flat-roofed structure offers additional facilities. After crossing a section of the paved parking lot, the path slips through a grove of cedars, turns toward the shoreline, then joins a paved surface for a short distance.

At the 0.8-mile mark, it merges at the side of the park's access road and follows it for much of the remaining distance. The beach and its crashing waves lie closeby but sand dunes block the view. After turning into a final area of dunes and grasses, the bike path ends near the **Meigs Point** parking lot and beach house.

Willard's Island offers a worthwhile, 0.8-mile loop from the Meigs Point area. Used as a campground until 1972, this acreage has been reclaimed by dense foliage and the old paved roads which once accessed the campsites now serve as a nature trail. Follow the driveway that runs behind the **nature center** to a gate at the northern edge of a mowed field, where the trail begins. A wooden viewing platform at the north end of the island offers a look at **Dudley Creek**, the mouth of the **Hammonassett River**, and surrounding marshland.

Currently under construction, the nearby **Shoreline Greenway Tr.** will invite bicyclists and foot travelers into the

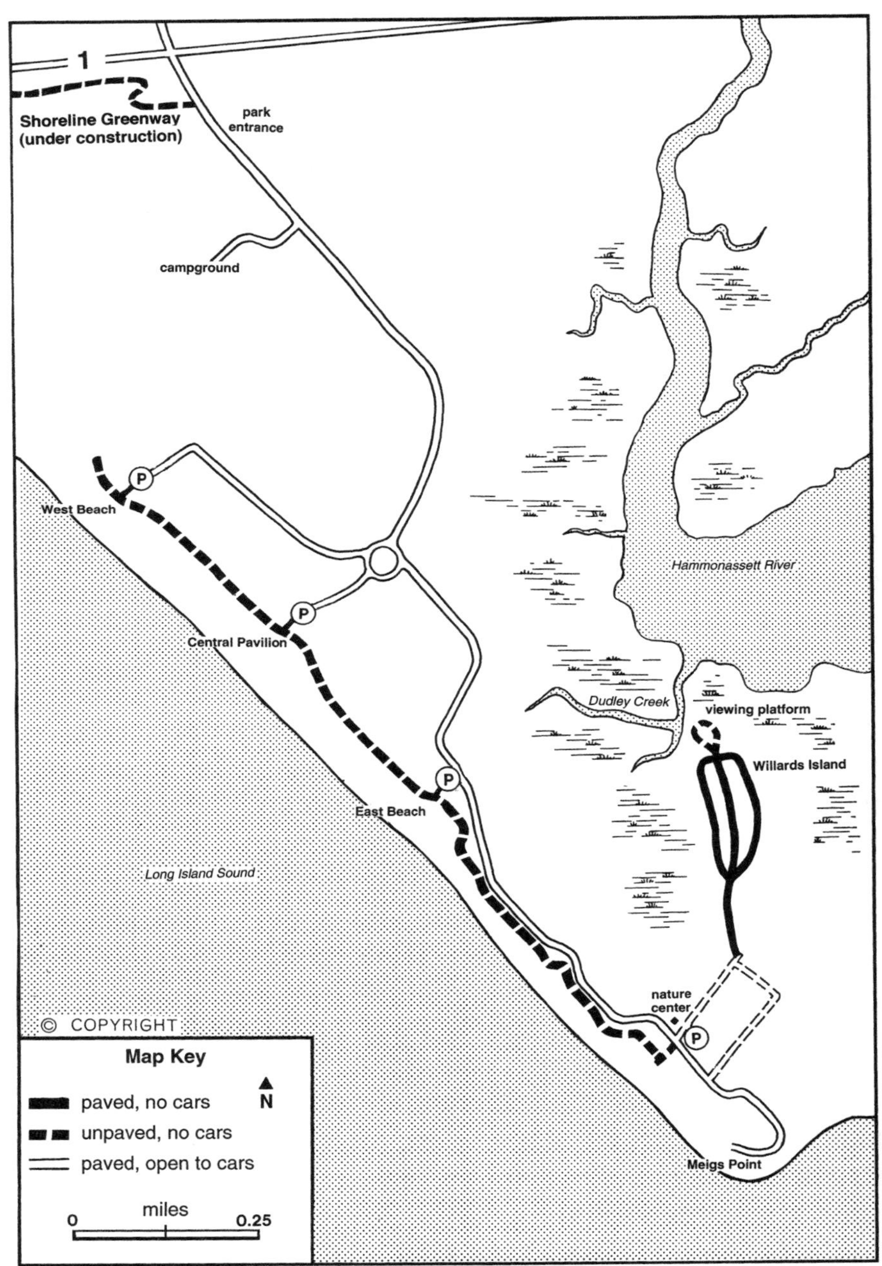
1
Shoreline Greenway
(under construction)
park
entrance
campground
West Beach
Central Pavilion
East Beach
Long Island Sound
Hammonassett River
Dudley Creek
viewing platform
Willards Island
nature
center
Meigs Point
P
© COPYRIGHT
Map Key
paved, no cars
unpaved, no cars
paved, open to cars
N
miles
0
0.25

shade of woods. Open marshland along the way allows several good views. The trail's smooth, stone dust surface will eventually extend west from the park's entrance drive for a mile to Webster Point Rd., paralleling **Rte. 1** as it rolls with small slopes and turns through trees and a few stone walls. The greenway is destined to be a 25-mile route stretching from Hammonassett State Park to New Haven Harbor.

BACKGROUND:

Hammonassett, a Native American word meaning *"where we dig holes in the ground,"* was settled by Europeans in the late 1630's and supported a small agricultural and fishing community for a few hundred years. Settlers processed fish for fertilizer and oil, harvested salt hay from the marshes, and grew potatoes and wheat in the fields. In the late 1890's a local arms manufacturer used the peninsula as a rifle range.

Hammonassett Beach State Park was established in 1919 when the first parcels of land were acquired by the state. The park officially opened in 1920 and quickly became a popular attraction for growing numbers of summer vacationers who arrived by car from distant places and camped beside the shore. Colonies of summer cottages sprouted near the park during this period. Today, Hammonassett's campground holds a huge capacity and its 2-mile beach draws thousands of visitors on peak days, making it one of Connecticut's most popular parks.

DRIVING DIRECTIONS:

From I-95 take Exit 62 and drive south for 1.3 miles on the Hammonassett Connector to a traffic signal at Rte. 1. Continue straight through the intersection to the park's entrance gate, and park in the lots shown on the map.

TOILETS:

at the beach access points during the swimming season

ADDITIONAL INFORMATION:

Hammonassett Beach State Park, Box 271, Madison, CT 06443, (203) 245-2785
Campground: (203) 245-1817
Shoreline Greenway, www.shorelinegreenwaytrail.org

30 Hop River State Park Trail

Manchester - Coventry, CT

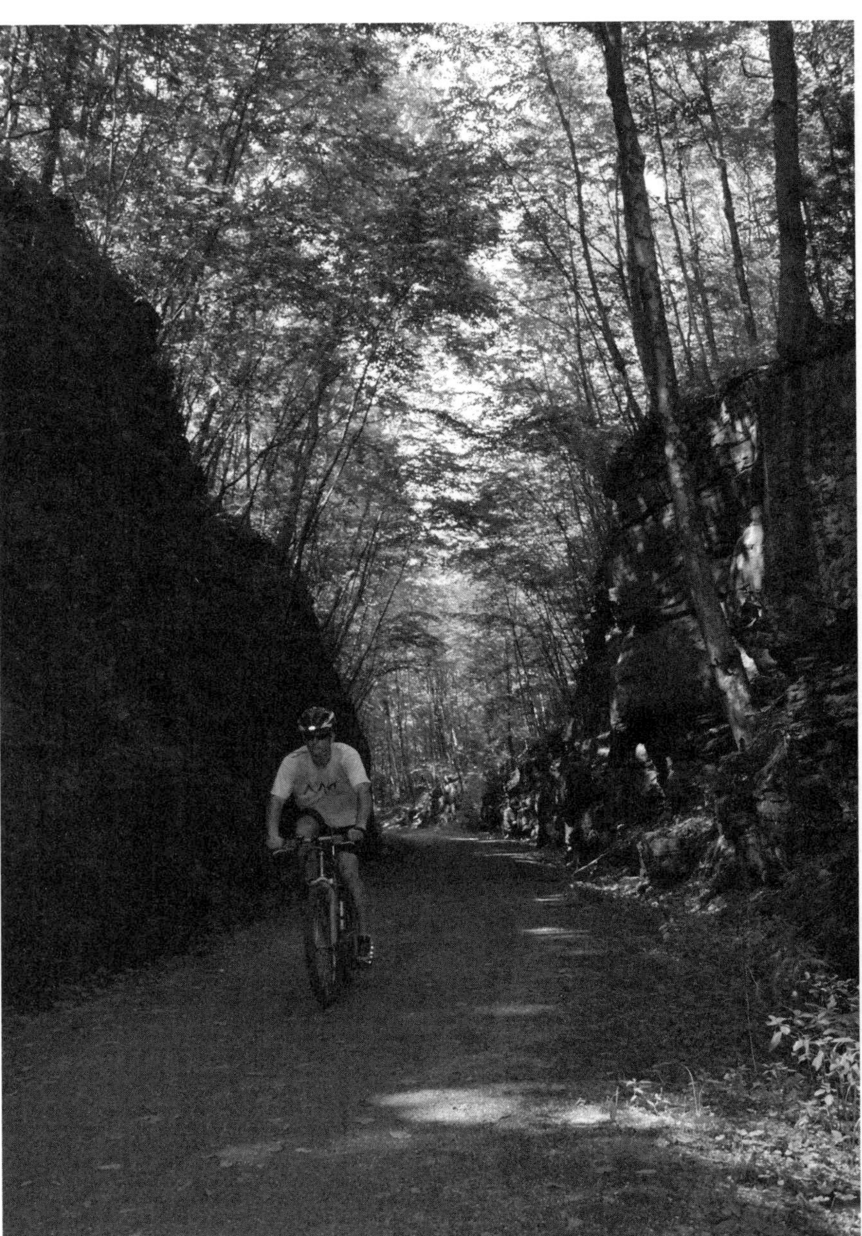

LENGTH: 19.2 miles, plus a 3.4-mile spur to Rockville
SURFACE: mostly stone dust, some crushed stone and dirt
TERRAIN: gradual slopes

This rail-trail connects the Manchester and Willimantic areas with a woodsy route through Bolton Notch and smooth riding past forested hillsides, isolated farm fields, and the peaceful flow of the Hop River.

RULES & SAFETY:

• Bicyclists should yield to pedestrians.

• Keep to the right, pass on the left, and alert others (*"On your left..."*) when approaching from behind to avoid startling them.

• Ride at a safe speed, and use extra caution when children and pets are present since their movements can be unpredictable.

• When encountering horses, make verbal contact with the rider and be ready to stop at the side of the trail.

• Be self-sufficient with food, water, and bike repair supplies since the trail reaches remote areas.

• Hunting occurs in the area, mostly in the late fall (except on Sundays, when it's prohibited by state law); wear an article of blaze orange clothing during this time.

• Be careful not to block trailhead gates when parking.

• The trail is open from sunrise to sunset.

ORIENTATION:

The Hop River State Park Tr. has a mostly east-west orientation and extends from Manchester at the western terminus through Vernon, Bolton, Andover, Columbia, and Coventry. Trailhead parking lots exist along the western portion of the trail in Manchester, Vernon, and Bolton Notch, and smaller spaces for parking are available at many of the trail/road intersections along the eastern portion.

Overall trail conditions tend to be best along the western portion of the trail which has a smooth surface of stone dust, crosswalks at road intersections, benches, and other amenities. This section also gets the most use.

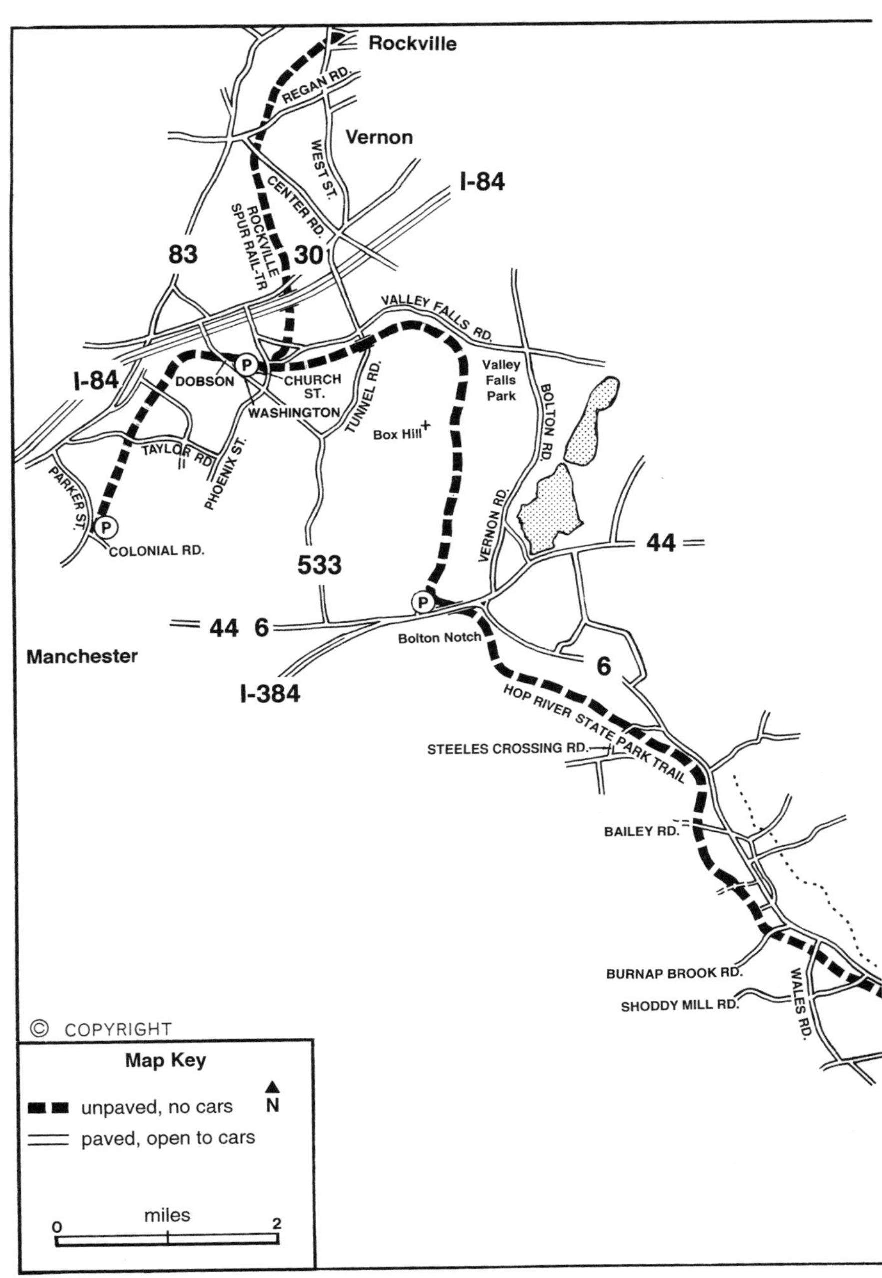
Rockville
REGAN RD.
Vernon
WEST ST.
I-84
CENTER RD.
ROCKVILLE SPUR RAIL-TR
83
30
VALLEY FALLS RD.
Valley Falls Park
I-84
DOBSON
CHURCH ST.
WASHINGTON
TUNNEL RD.
BOLTON RD.
Box Hill
TAYLOR RD
PHOENIX ST.
PARKER ST.
VERNON RD.
COLONIAL RD.
44
533
44 6
Bolton Notch
Manchester
6
I-384
HOP RIVER STATE PARK TRAIL
STEELES CROSSING RD.
BAILEY RD.
BURNAP BROOK RD.
SHODDY MILL RD.
WALES RD.
© COPYRIGHT
Map Key
unpaved, no cars
paved, open to cars
N
miles
0
2

Scenery is good along the entire trail but best on the approaches to Bolton Notch and in the flatter terrain along the Hop River. Trailhead gates block vehicle entry and sometimes display the names of intersecting roads, a useful aid when determining locations on the map.

Elevation changes are significant on the western half and minor on the eastern half, with the trail's highest point being Bolton Notch and the lowest being the endpoints in Manchester and Coventry. When starting from the high elevation of the Bolton Notch trailhead, remember that extra energy will be required for the uphill return leg of your ride.

TRAIL DESCRIPTION:

Beginning at the western endpoint at the **Colonial Rd.** trailhead in Manchester, the Hop River State Park Tr. heads north from a commercial/industrial area into the shade of woods. The trail passes residential neighborhoods and crosses the Vernon town line before intersecting **Taylor St.** where a slight incline develops, then crosses **Elm Hill Rd.** (1.4 miles) and rounds the side of a hill heading east. Cross-

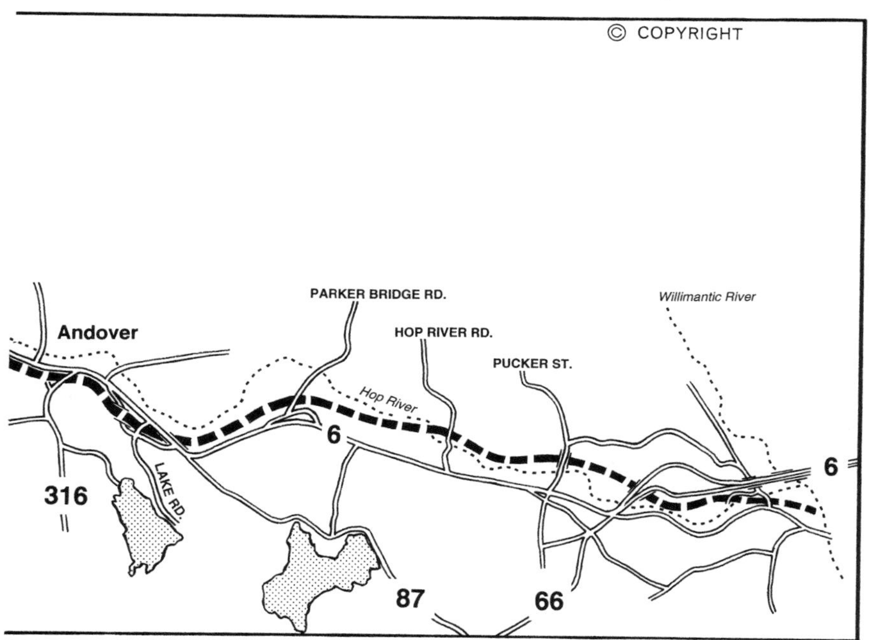

ing Dobson Rd., it parallels **Church St.** and reaches the Vernon trailhead (2.4 miles), site of the former Vernon Depot.

It descends abruptly at a missing bridge over Phoenix St. (2.5 miles) where the 3.4-mile **Rockville Spur Rail-Trail** branches to the left (north). Starting as a sidewalk along Warren Ave., this stone dust path crosses the road and enters woods with a downslope for the first half and uphill for the second half to the village of **Rockville**. It descends to the Tankerhoosen River, passes under **I-84**, and intersects five other roads along the way including busy **Rte. 30**.

The Hop River State Park Tr. continues east from Phoenix St. with an incline which lasts for the next 4 miles. It follows the top of a long, earthen causeway over **Tunnel Rd.** (3.3 miles), named for its one-lane passageway under the rail bed, then turns south in a broad curve to the right and climbs at a more noticeable pace along the side of **Box Hill**. Outcroppings of ledge loom above the trail on one side as the valley of Railroad Brook falls away on the other. At 5.8 miles, the trail hits the Bolton town line as the stream valley tightens to a narrow gap.

The **Bolton Notch** trailhead appears at the 6.8-mile mark and also serves a boat launch for Bolton Notch Pond on the right. Just ahead, the trail turns through the arched bridge of **Rte. 6/Rte. 44** and continues below ground level for a half-mile in a cut blasted into the top of the notch.

It descends from this high point for most of the remaining distance, turning with the contours of a forested slope and showing few signs of civilization for the next few miles. The trail intersects **Steel Crossing Rd.** (8.9 miles), briefly enters the town of Coventry, then crosses the Andover line before the intersection of **Bailey Rd.** (10.1 miles). The stone dust surface lasts until **Burnap Brook Rd.** (11.3 miles) and conditions degrade to hard-packed gravel and dirt as the trail approaches Andover center.

A bridge carries it over **Rte. 316** (13.0 miles) as the slope flattens and the trail turns eastward. After crossing **Lake Rd.**, it enters a long tunnel under Rte. 6 (14.0 miles) and then joins the course of the peaceful **Hop River** for its remaining miles and enjoys many scenic views along the way. It reaches the Columbia town line at **Parker Bridge Rd.** (15.3 miles) where a stone dust surface returns for the next 1.2 miles to a bridge over the river at the Coventry line.

Just beyond this, it intersects **Hop River Rd.** (16.7 miles). The next mile offers more nice scenery of the river, a few hay fields, and the shade of quiet woods but also a bumpier ride from horse hoof prints. Narrowing slightly, the trail travels under **Pucker St.** (17.8 miles), under two bridges carrying Rte. 6, and under a set of powerlines before ending at **Kings Rd.**, 19.2 miles from the Manchester terminus.

BACKGROUND:

The Hop River State Park Tr. follows the former Hartford, Providence, and Fishkill Railroad which was built in 1854. For about 100 years, it provided a direct connection between the Connecticut and Rhode Island capitols as well as a valuable transportation link for the many small towns along the route.

The state's Dept. of Environmental Protection acquired the line in 1987 for recreational use and the trail has been developed in stages since that time. With help from the national guard in 1995, the Vernon section was the first to be improved and future work is planned along the less-developed sections. The trail forms a leg of the East Coast Greenway, a 2600-mile route from Maine to Florida.

DRIVING DIRECTIONS:

Colonial Rd. trailhead: From I-84 take Exit 64 and follow signs for Rte. 83 south. Continue on Rte. 83 south for 1 mile from the interstate overpass. Turn left on Parker St. and drive for 0.9 miles, turn left on Colonial Rd., then left into the parking lot.

Bolton Notch trailhead: From I-384 drive to the eastern end of the highway, fork left on Rte. 44 east, then turn left and reverse direction at signs for Rte. 44 west. Continue on Rte. 44 west for less than a half-mile and turn right on a narrow road at a *"boat launch"* sign. Park at the end.

TOILETS:

Vernon trailhead (in season)

ADDITIONAL INFORMATION:

Connecticut Dept. of Environmental Protection, www.ct.gov/dep

31 Airline State Park Trail

East Hampton - Lebanon, CT

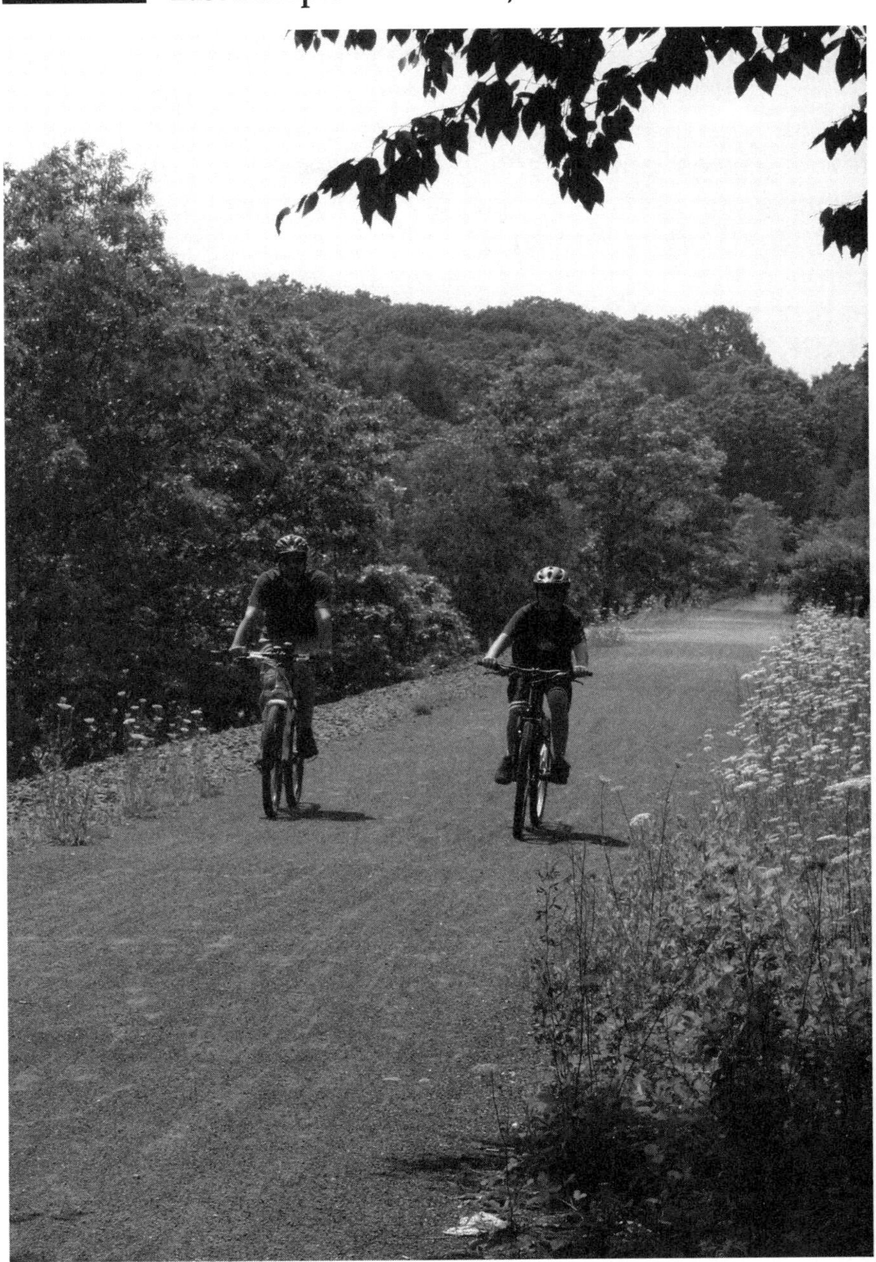

LENGTH: 20.0 miles
SURFACE: stone dust
TERRAIN: gradual slopes

Spanning eastern Connecticut, the 3-part Airline State Park Trail defies surrounding hills and valleys with long, slow turns and gentle slopes. This southern leg of the trail offers a firm, smooth surface and easy rolling through miles of deep woods.

RULES & SAFETY:

• Keep to the right, pass on the left, and alert others (*"On your left..."*) when approaching from behind.

• The trail reaches remote areas so be self-sufficient with food, water, and bike repair supplies.

• At road intersections, stop and look both ways before crossing and assume that drivers do not see you.

• When encountering horses, bicyclists should stop at the side of the trail and make verbal contact with the rider so that the animal will feel safe.

• Hunting is permitted along much of the trail (although it is prohibited by state law on Sundays). If possible, wear blaze orange clothing between mid-October and late December, the most popular hunting season.

• Respect the private property along the trail.

• Be careful not to block trailhead gates when parking since work crews and emergency vehicles need access.

• Dogs must be leashed and their wastes removed.

• Motorized vehicles are prohibited.

• The trail is open from sunrise to sunset.

ORIENTATION:

This description covers the southern leg of the Airline State Park Trail from East Hampton in the southwest to Lebanon in the northeast. Other portions of the Airline State Park Trail are detailed in chapters 32 and 33.

This section of the trail offers a consistent, 10-foot-wide surface of stone dust with cleared shoulders. Two detours from the original rail bed include a brief loop under a

Rte 2 bridge in Colchester, and a longer, hillier on-road route at Cooks Hill Rd. in Lebanon.

The trail's elevation profile has the lowest point at the crossing of the Salmon River in Colchester and another low point at the Willimantic River (eastern terminus) in Lebanon. The highest point is Leonard Bridge Rd. in Lebanon and another high point is the Smith St. trailhead (near the western terminus). Remember that starting a ride from a high point will require an uphill effort when returning.

Trailhead parking lots are located at Smith St. in East Hampton, Rte. 2 (Exit 16) in Colchester, and Rte. 85 in Hebron. Smaller, roadside spots are present at many other trail/road intersections. Benches and picnic tables await at points along the way and mileage markers, originating at the southwestern end, allow travelers to measure their progress. In general, the trail's southwestern half holds the most notable scenery and gets the most usage while its northeastern half has lots of woods and gets less usage.

TRAIL DESCRIPTION:

Begin at the East Hampton trailhead on **Smith St.** To the southwest (across the street from the parking lot), the Airline State Park Trail runs for a half-mile downhill to **Watrous St.** near **East Hampton** center.

To the northeast (past the trailhead sign), the trail extends for 19.5 miles. Starting with a broad, righthand turn toward the southeast, the trail develops a faint downhill slope which lasts for most of the next 4.7 miles, allowing an easy start but requiring extra effort on the return ride.

At 1.3 miles it passes through a long cut in the bedrock of a hill and emerges at the start of the **Rapallo Viaduct**, a high, quarter-mile-long earthen causeway. Named for a railroad director, it was originally a 60-foot-tall bridge built over **Flat Brook** in 1873 but was filled in 1913 in order to accommodate heavier trains. Steel portions of the original bridge protrude at points along the trail surface. The viaduct provides an excellent view over a wetland to the north but visitors are urged to use appropriate caution along its high, steep bankings.

The trail returns to woods on the other side and soon enters **Salmon River State Forest**, a 6115-acre preserve which is popular for hunting and fishing. The property offers good scenery along the next few miles of the trail.

Near the 2.3-mile mark the trail turns to the east, crosses the Colchester town line, and approaches the **Lyman Viaduct** at the 2.6-mile mark. Named after the railroad's first president, this larger viaduct also originated as a bridge in 1873 and was filled in 1913 to accommodate heavier trains. Parts of the original steel structure remain visible above the fill as reminders of the huge bridge now buried in gravel. The trail surface stands about 140 feet above **Dickinson Brook** at the bottom of the valley and allows unbroken views to the north and south.

The Airline reaches a small parking area at a sharp, hairpin turn on **Bull Hill Rd.** after 3.1 miles. Turning northeasterly, it is confined to a shelf along a slope as it gently descends through cuts and fills in the narrow valley of the **Salmon River**. Walls of exposed bedrock and the evergreen foliage of mountain laurel line the edges. **River Rd.**, barely visible through the forest, parallels at a lower elevation and passes through a stone arch bridge underneath the trail at the 4.7-mile mark.

A bridge carries the Airline Trail high over the Salmon River shortly beyond this and the trail leaves the state forest heading east on a mile-long straightaway. A slight uphill grade develops at this point. The trail crosses River Rd. again at the 5.5-mile mark, turns back to the northeast at the intersection of **Rte. 149** (6.0 miles), then emerges a *Park & Ride* lot beside **Rte. 2** (**Exit 16**) (6.4-miles).

Here the trail takes a brief, on-road detour because the original rail bed has been obstructed by the highway. Exiting the parking lot, turn right on Rte. 149 and pass under Rte. 2, then look for the trail resuming on the right. It follows the highway's embankment for a short distance before rejoining the original railroad grade.

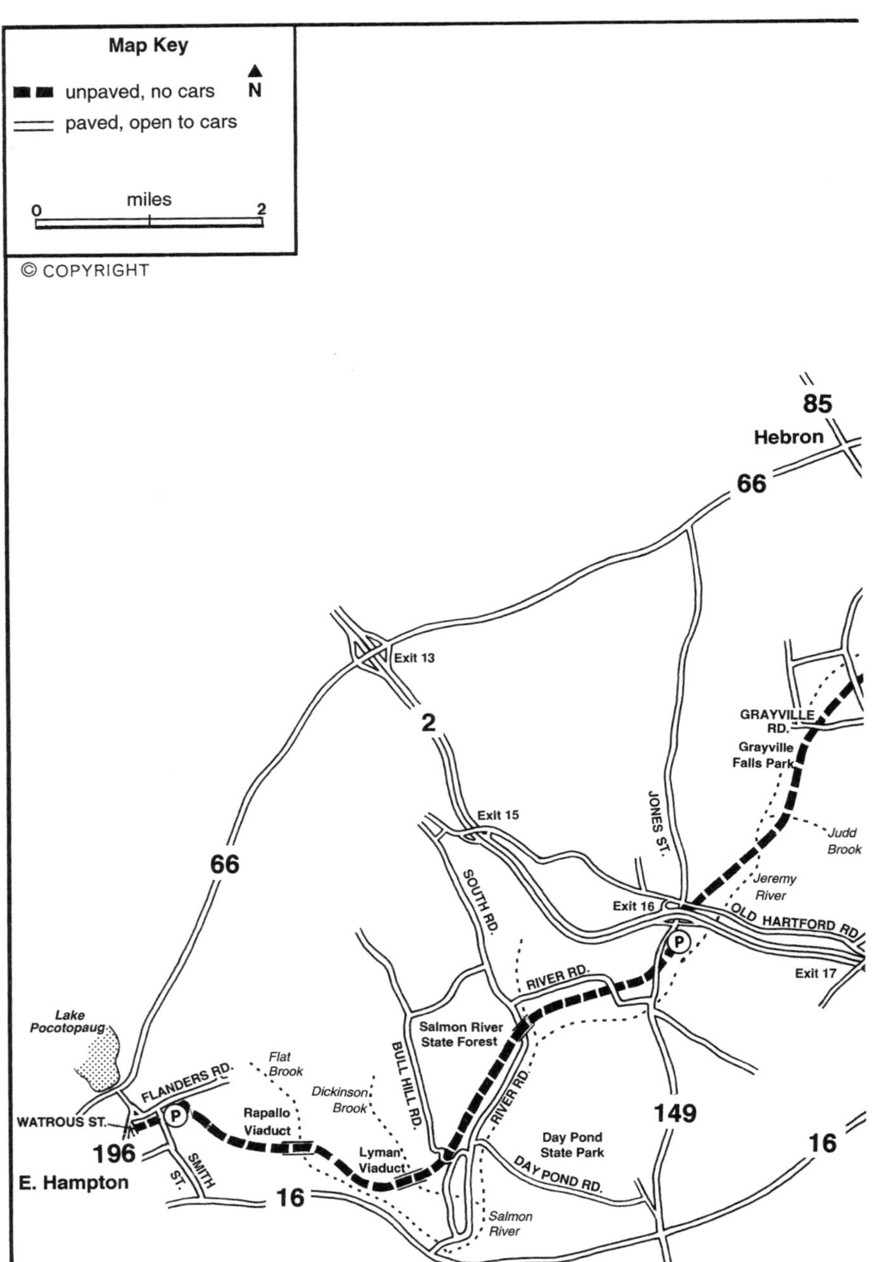

Map Key
unpaved, no cars
paved, open to cars
N
miles
0
2
© COPYRIGHT
85
Hebron
66
Exit 13
2
GRAYVILLE RD.
Grayville Falls Park
Exit 15
JONES ST.
Judd Brook
66
SOUTH RD.
Jeremy River
Exit 16
OLD HARTFORD RD.
Exit 17
RIVER RD.
Salmon River State Forest
Lake Pocotopaug
Flat Brook
FLANDERS RD.
Dickinson Brook
BULL HILL RD.
RIVER RD.
Rapallo Viaduct
149
WATROUS ST.
Day Pond State Park
16
196
Lyman Viaduct
SMITH ST.
DAY POND RD.
E. Hampton
16
Salmon River

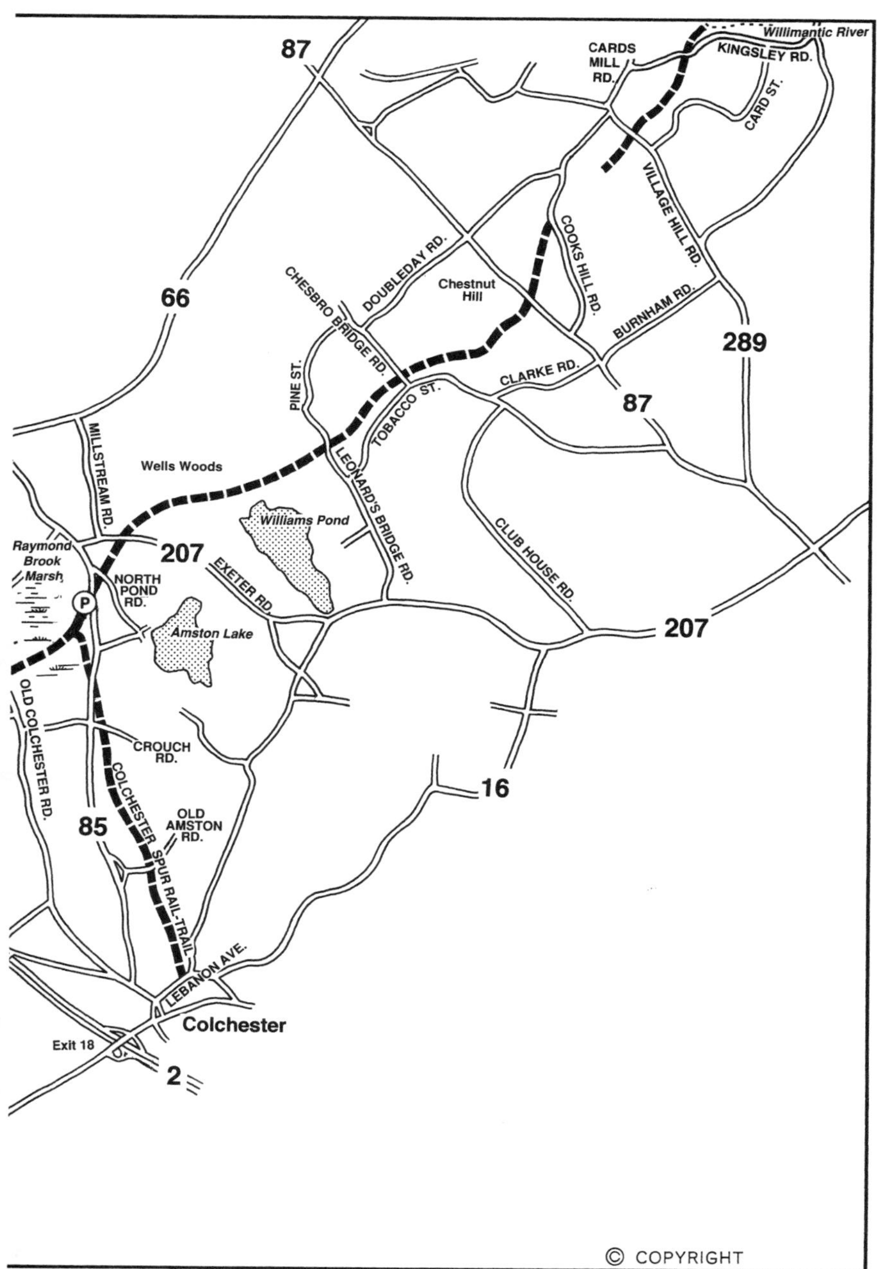
87
CARDS
MILL
RD.
Willimantic River
KINGSLEY RD.
CARD ST.
VILLAGE HILL RD.
COOKS HILL RD.
DOUBLEDAY RD.
Chestnut
Hill
CHESBRO BRIDGE RD.
66
BURNHAM RD.
289
PINE ST.
CLARKE RD.
87
TOBACCO ST.
MILLSTREAM RD.
Wells Woods
LEONARD'S BRIDGE RD.
Williams Pond
CLUB HOUSE RD.
Raymond
Brook
Marsh
207
NORTH
POND
RD.
EXETER RD.
P
Amston Lake
207
OLD COLCHESTER RD.
CROUCH
RD.
16
COLCHESTER SPUR RAIL-TRAIL
85
OLD
AMSTON
RD.
LEBANON AVE.
Colchester
Exit 18
2
© COPYRIGHT

A small trailhead marks the intersection of **Old Hartford Rd.** (6.7 miles). The trail extends over a mostly flat, straight course for almost a mile to a bridge over **Jeremy River** (7.6 miles) then tilts upward on a slight slope as it turns north, crosses **Judd Brook**, and enters the town of Hebron. A straight, mile-long uphill grade brings the trail through **Grayville Falls Park**, a town-owned preserve.

The trail flattens at **Grayville Rd.** (8.9 miles) and follows a corridor of trees for the next half-mile to **Old Colchester Rd.** Young hardwoods have encroached along the shoulders of this stretch giving it a narrower feel even though the prepared surface remains wide.

The next 1.2 miles ranks among the Airline's most scenic. The trail emerges from forest at **Raymond Brook Marsh**, a vast wetland with an expansive view, traverses it on a half-mile-long causeway, and then returns to tree cover for the last half-mile to **Rte. 85** (10.7 miles).

Look for the **Colchester Spur Rail-Trail** branching on the right just before Rte. 85. This 3.4-mile trail runs south, paralleling Rte. 85 and crossing several side roads before ending near **Colchester** center at the former railroad station on **Lebanon Ave.** Its surface starts with stone dust but currently degrades to gravel along the southernmost portion.

Continuing northeastward, the Airline Trail crosses Rte. 85, **North Pond Rd.**, and **Exeter Rd.** (**Rte. 207**) in the next 0.6 miles. All three intersections deserve extra caution as a result of high traffic speeds, slopes, and poor visibility. Crosswalks and signs are in place to assist trail travelers.

The next 2.1-mile leg to **Leonard Bridge Rd.** begins in the open scenery of another marsh, enters the town of Lebanon and the shade of **Wells Woods**, and rises on an incline to the trail's highest point. A gentle downslope ensues after Leonard Bridge Rd. (13.4 miles), where the bridge no longer stands and trail users must climb a slope in order to cross the street. A mile ahead, the same is true at **Chesbro Bridge Rd.** (14.4 miles). Continuing downward on a faint slope, the trail meets the side of **Chestnut Hill** with a series of cuts and fills, crosses **Trumbull Hwy.** (**Rte. 87**) (15.9 miles), then straightens to **Cooks Hill Rd.** (16.6 miles).

Future development will continue the trail straight at this point but currently a detour on hilly back roads is required. Turn left (north) on Cooks Hill Rd. and ride for 1.2 miles to the end at the bottom of a steep slope, turn right (south) on **Valley Hill Rd.** and ride for another quarter-mile, then look for the trail resuming on the left side (18.1-miles).

Continuing northeastward, the trail descends gradually. After a mile, it rises on a bank to cross **Kingsley Rd.** (19.1 miles) at the site of another filled bridge and runs for a final 0.4 miles before ending at the **Willimantic River**, 19.5 miles from the Smith St. trailhead in E. Hampton.

BACKGROUND:

The trail follows the route of the Air Line Railroad, built in 1873 along an "air-line" route between New York and Boston. Since it bypassed Connecticut's capitol, construction of such a direct line faced political controversy as well as natural obstacles including a crossing of the Connecticut River and a difficult topography. The Air Line's relatively hilly, curvy profile eventually restricted its success as trailns began to carry heavier loads and opted for flatter routes. A 1955 flood destroyed the railroad's bridge over the Quinebaug River in Putnam and it was never rebuilt.

The Connecticut Dept. of Environmental Protection (D.E.P.) acquired the railbed as a linear park in 1996. With the help of federal funding, the D.E.P. and town crews began clearing trees and debris, refurbishing bridges, and laying the stone dust surface.

DRIVING DIRECTIONS:

Smith St., East Hampton trailhead: From Rte. 2, take Exit 13 and follow Rte. 66 west for 4.2 miles. Turn left on Rte. 196 south and drive for 0.4 miles, then turn left on Flanders Rd. Continue for a quarter-mile, turn right on Smith St., and find the trailhead a short distance ahead on the left.

Rte. 85, Hebron trailhead: From Rte. 2, take Exit 18 and follow Rte. 16 east for 0.4 miles. Turn left on Rte. 85 north and continue for 4.1 miles to the trailhead on the left.

TOILETS:

none on-site

ADDITIONAL INFORMATION:

Connecticut Dept. of Environmental Protection, www.ct.gov/dep

32 Airline State Park Trail

Windham - Putnam, CT

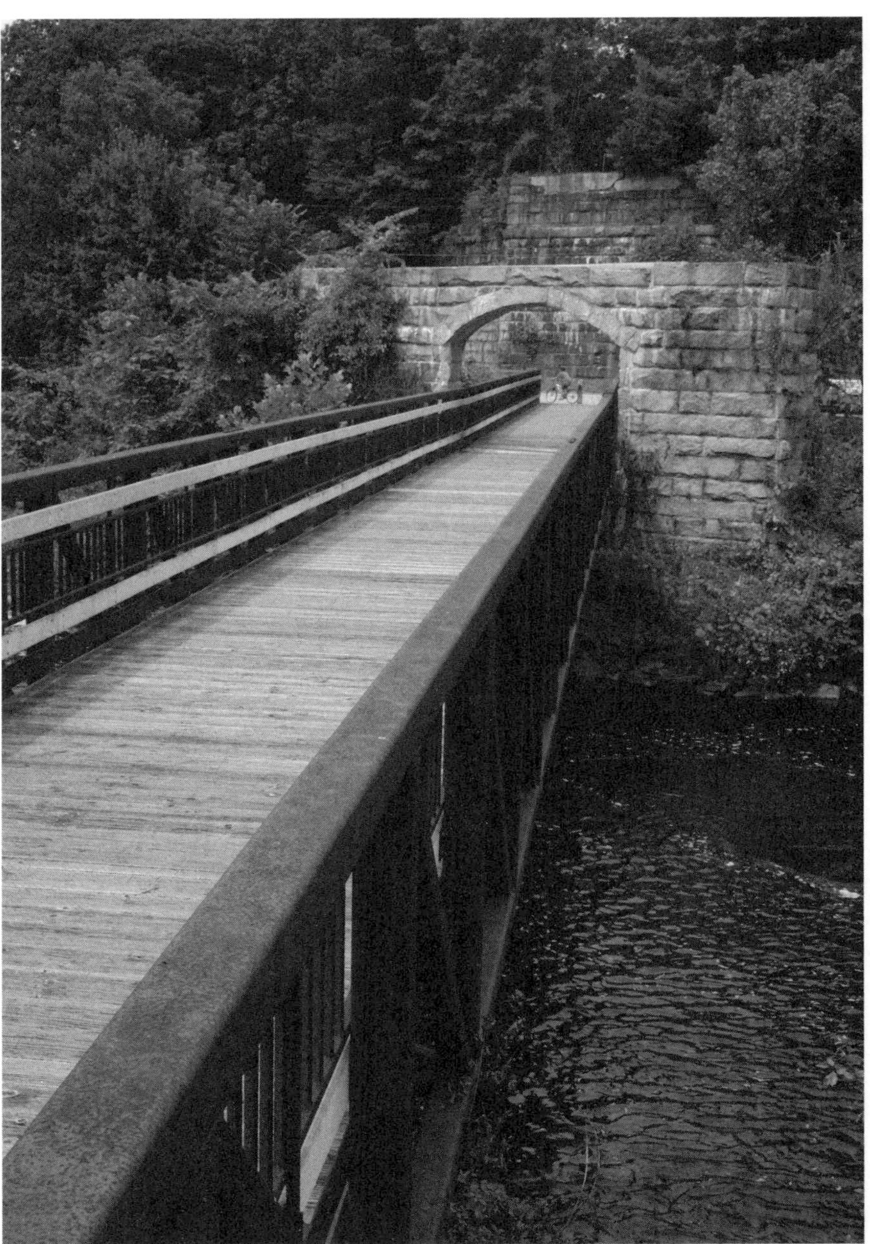

LENGTH: 24.5 miles, plus 1.2-mile side trail
SURFACE: varies between paved, processed stone, and dirt
TERRAIN: gentle, with slopes at detours from the rail line
NOTE: wide-tired bikes are advised

This midsection of the Airline connects Willimantic with Putnam through rural farmland and forests. Most of it has a rideable, gravelly surface but some rougher areas require a mountain bike.

RULES & SAFETY:

• Keep to the right, pass on the left, and alert others (*"On your left..."*) when approaching from behind.

• The trail reaches remote areas so be self-sufficient with food, water, and bike repair supplies.

• At road intersections, stop and look both ways before crossing and assume that drivers do not see you.

• When approaching horses, bicyclists should stop and make verbal contact with the rider so the animal feels safe.

• Hunting is permitted along much of the trail (although it is prohibited by state law on Sundays). If possible, wear blaze orange clothing during hunting season in late fall.

• Respect the private property along the trail.

• Be careful not to block trailhead gates when parking since work crews and emergency vehicles need access.

• Pets must be leashed and their wastes removed.

• Motorized vehicles are prohibited.

• The trail is open from sunrise to sunset.

ORIENTATION:

This description covers the Airline State Park Trail from Willimantic (in Windham) in the southwest to Putnam in the northeast, and includes the adjoining Putnam River Tr. Other sections are detailed in chapters 31 and 33.

The trail surface varies widely. At the southwest end in Willimantic, 2.4 miles of paved trail allow easy biking. Most of the remaining distance has not been formally developed but its surface of processed stone or gravel, while bumpy in places, is suitable for wide-tired bicycles. Loose, eroded, or poorly drained areas occur along the northeastern portion of the trail and are best ridden with a mountain bike.

Trailheads include those shown on the map as well as gravel turnouts at several trail/road intersections. Gates block vehicles from entering but signs, crosswalks, and other amenities do not exist along most of the trail.

The highest elevation is near the midpoint at Station Rd. in Hampton and the lowest elevations are the endpoints in Willimantic and Putnam.

TRAIL DESCRIPTION:

Begin at the southwest endpoint in Willimantic (in the town of Windham) near the intersection of **Jackson St.** and Union St. Follow the sidewalk heading northeast along the parking lot to Milk St. to reach the trail which starts with a paved surface in a residential area. The Airline intersects **Ash St.** after three quarters of a mile, crosses a bridge over the **Natchaug River** (1 mile), and extends on a straight-line course through a mixed retail and industrial area.

Near the intersection of **Rte. 66** (1.9 miles), the trail detours from the rail corridor where highway off-ramps have been built. It climbs a noticeable slope beside **Tuckie Rd.** then descends beside an exit ramp back to the rail bed, where the paved surface reverts to stone dust for the next few miles. A gentle downslope carries the trail through woods to the **Windham Atlantic White Cedar Bog** which opens the scenery on both sides.

The trail descends a banking at a missing bridge over **Rte. 203** (3.8 miles) then scrambles up the opposite side. A wooden bridge spans **Boulevard Rd.** (4.0 miles) before the trail hits the Chaplin town line, loses the stone dust surface for a dirt/gravel finish, and turns to the right (east) paralleling **Lynch Rd.** at the foot of **Beaver Hill**. The curve reverses back to the left (north) at **Chewink Rd.** (6.0 miles) where another missing bridge creates short slopes for the trail.

The next two miles are woodsy and cross a high causeway over a stream before hitting the Hampton town line and **S. Brook Rd.** (7.9 miles). Crushed stone forms a smooth surface for much of the next mile as the trail continues under **Rte. 6** (8.3 miles) and intersects **Potter Rd.** (8.9 miles) near the **Goodwin State Forest** trailhead.

Continuing, the trail rises on a mile-long straightaway heading north near **Pine Acres Lake**. It makes a brief descent to the crossing of **Estabrooks Rd.** (10.4 miles), climbs back to the railbed, and turns eastward on another causeway built through a low-lying area. An even surface of crushed stone and gravel allows smooth rolling here.

The uphill pitch flattens as the trail enters an area of marshland and reaches its highest elevation at **Station Rd.** (11.7 miles) where a clearing and cluster of houses mark the former railroad stop known as **Rawson**.

Turning northward again, the trail returns to woods with a slight downslope that lasts for most of the remaining distance. After a causeway over Hampton Brook, it curves to the northeast at the intersection of **Griffin Rd.** (12.7 miles) and straightens for the next mile and a half, passing the southern shore of **Hampton Reservoir** near **Kenyon Rd.** (13.2 miles) and several farm fields on the way to **Lewis Rd.** (14.1 miles), where the rail bed has been filled and trail users must scramble up a banking.

The riding gets rougher over much of the remaining distance with overgrown conditions, bumpy surfaces, and poor drainage in some places. The next 1.3 miles have a few wet spots as the trail enters Pomfret and intersects **Rte. 97** (15.4 miles), then a grassy third of a mile extends to **Brooklyn Rd.** (15.7 miles) where an inscribed rock marks the former train stop of **Elliot Station**.

The trail bends left at the base of **Easter Hill** and heads north along its rocky slope on a 2-mile leg through forest and wetland to the first crossing of Rte. 44 (17.7 miles). Curving back to the east, the next mile hits both **Osgood Rd.** and **Babbit Hill Rd.** at former bridge sites which have been filled, requiring short climbs at each. The second crossing of Rte. 44 (20.1 miles) occurs just beyond the former **Pomfret Station**, now a developed trailhead with a

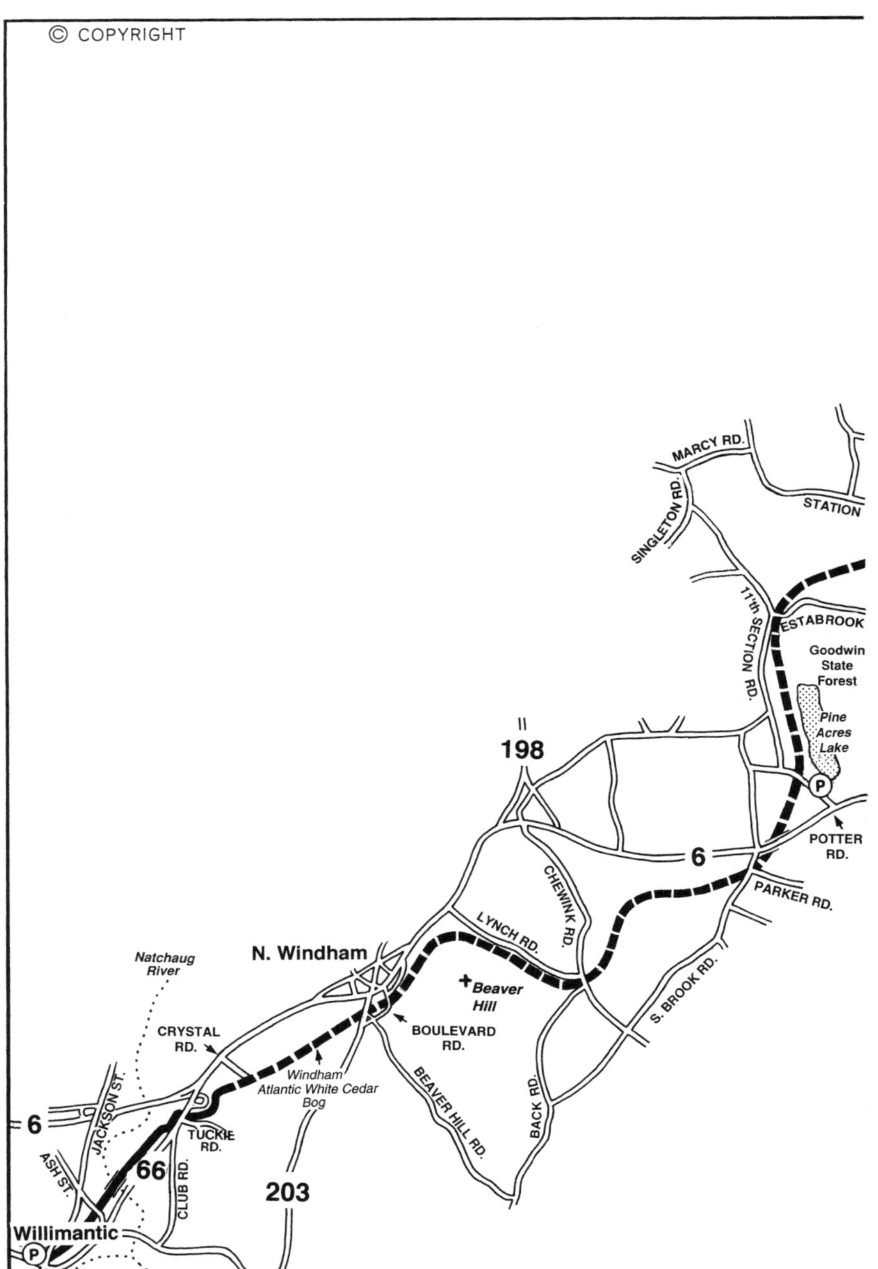

MARCY RD.
SINGLETON RD.
STATION
11'th SECTION RD.
ESTABROOK
Goodwin State Forest
Pine Acres Lake
198
P
POTTER RD.
6
PARKER RD.
CHEWINK RD.
LYNCH RD.
N. Windham
Natchaug River
Beaver Hill
S. BROOK RD.
BOULEVARD RD.
CRYSTAL RD.
Windham Atlantic White Cedar Bog
BEAVER HILL RD.
BACK RD.
JACKSON ST.
6
TUCKIE RD.
ASH ST.
66
CLUB RD.
203
Willimantic
P

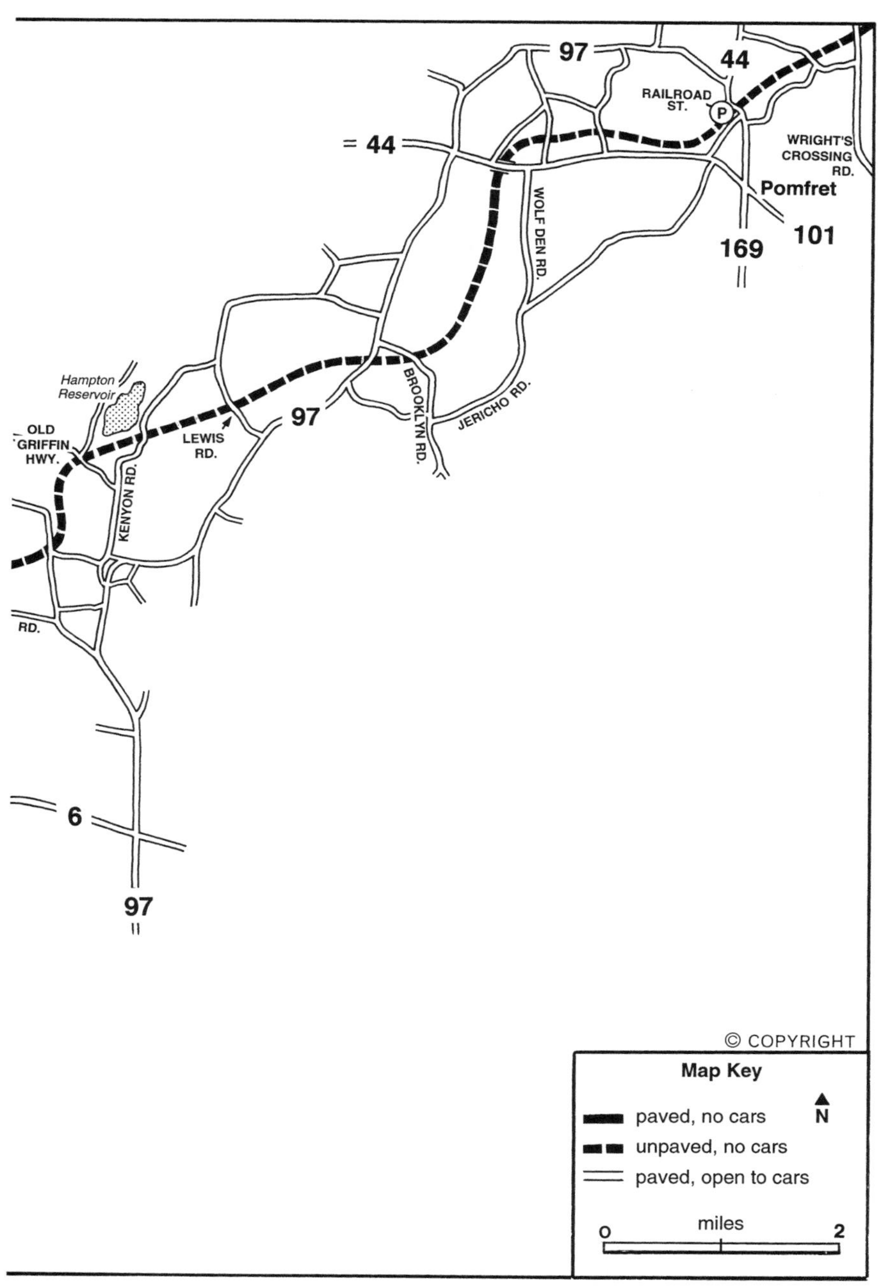
97
44
RAILROAD ST.
P
44
WRIGHT'S CROSSING RD.
Pomfret
WOLF DEN RD.
169
101
Hampton Reservoir
OLD GRIFFIN HWY.
LEWIS RD.
97
BROOKLYN RD.
JERICHO RD.
KENYON RD.
RD.
6
97
© COPYRIGHT
Map Key
N
paved, no cars
unpaved, no cars
paved, open to cars
miles
0
2

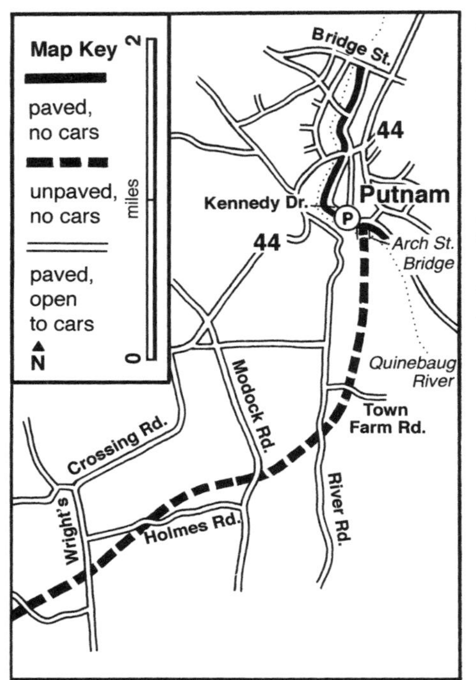

pavilion and historical display. Use caution when descending to the crosswalk at busy Rte. 44.

The treadway narrows but remains smooth for the next mile. The trail crosses a high causeway built across a wetland, drops abruptly at a missing bridge over **Needles Eye Rd.** (20.9 miles), and passes an Audubon sanctuary before **Wright's Crossing Rd.** (21.3 miles).

The Airline's last 2.7 miles have rideable conditions but a few rough spots and poorly drained areas are best handled with a mountain bike. A washout forces the trail off the rail bed before it crosses **Holmes Rd.** (21.8 miles) where it climbs and descends a filled bridge site. Crossing **Modock Rd.** (22.6 miles) at the Putnam town line, the trail passes through a long cut in a hill where puddles mire the surface, emerges on a high causeway built over a brook, then turns northward at the intersections of **River Rd.** (23.1 miles) and **Town Farm Rd.** (23.5 miles). The final mile has an eroded area but is an otherwise smooth ride along a causeway to the edge of the **Quinebaug River**, 24.5 miles from the Willimantic trailhead.

The railroad's original **Arch St. Bridge** is no longer intact but it is possible to descend the banking and cross the river on a rebuilt bike/pedestrian bridge to reach the **Putnam River Tr.**, a 1.2-mile paved pathway into downtown Putnam. Turn left on the opposite bank along **Kennedy Dr.** and follow it upstream through a landscaped strip of greenspace with shade trees, picnic tables, historical signs, and several trail-head parking lots. The highlight is just north of Rte. 44 where the trail offers a close view of the river tumbling off Cargill Falls.

BACKGROUND:

The trail follows the route of the Air Line Railroad, built in 1873 on an "air-line" between New York and Boston. Since it bypassed Connecticut's capitol, construction of this railroad faced political controversy as well as natural obstacles such as a crossing of the Connecticut River and a rough topography of hills and valleys. This hilly, curvy profile eventually restricted the Air Line's success as trains began to carry heavier loads and opted for flatter routes.

A severe hurricane in1955 caused a flood which destroyed the railroad's bridge over the Quinebaug River in Putnam and it was never replaced. Freight traffic on the remaining parts of the line eventually ceased and the state's Dept. of Environmental Protection acquired it for recreational use. It is now a designated part of the East Coast Greenway, a planned route from Maine to Florida.

DRIVING DIRECTIONS:

Willimantic from I-84: Take Exit 70 and follow Rte. 32 south for 15.9 miles. Turn left on Jackson St., immediately right on Union St., then left into the parking lot. Follow the sidewalk along the parking lot northeast to Milk St. to reach the trail.

Goodwin State Forest from I-395: Take Exit 91W and follow Rte. 6 west for 12.3 miles. Turn right on Potter Rd. and park in the lot ahead on the right. Follow Potter Rd. for another quarter-mile to reach the trail.

Pomfret Station from I-395: Take Exit 93 and follow Rte. 101 west for 4.4 miles. Turn right on Rte. 169 north and continue for 0.8 miles, then turn left on Railroad St. (just after the junction of Rte. 44). Parking is ahead on the left.

Putnam from I-395: Take Exit 95 and follow Kennedy Dr. north toward Putnam for about three quarters of a mile. Look for the parking lot on the left beside the river.

TOILETS:

Goodwin State Forest

ADDITIONAL INFORMATION:

Connecticut Dept. of Environmental Protection, www.ct.gov/dep

33 Airline State Park Trail S. New England Trunk Line Tr.

Thompson, CT - Franklin, MA

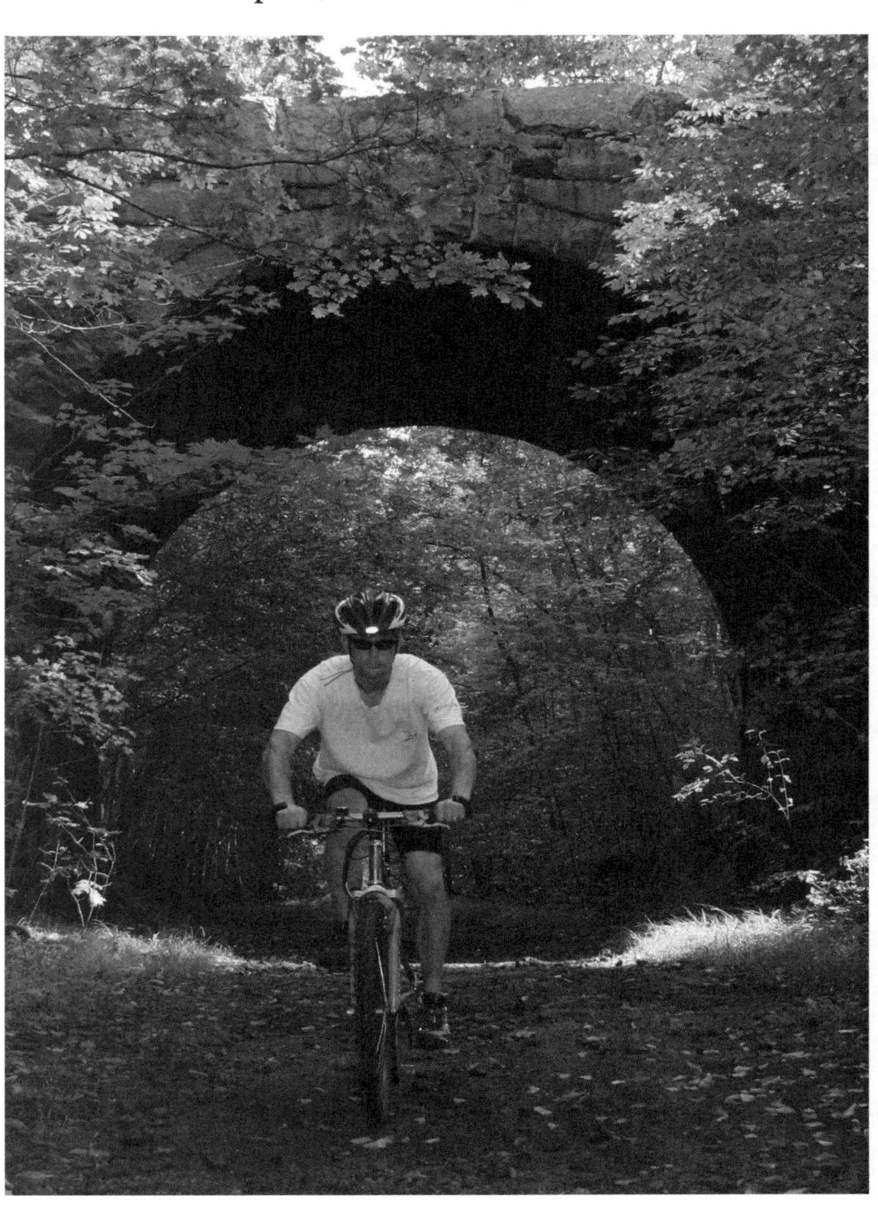

LENGTH: 25.7 miles, in 3 separate sections
SURFACE: gravel, rough in places
TERRAIN: gentle slopes
NOTE: mountain bikes advised

Joining the Southern New England Trunk Line Trail in Massachusetts, the Airline's northernmost leg has mostly rough riding, lots of overgrown areas, and several detours.

RULES & SAFETY:

• The trail reaches remote areas so be self-sufficient with food, water, and bike repair supplies.

• When encountering horses, bicyclists should stop at the side of the trail and make verbal contact with the rider so that the animal will feel safe.

• Hunting is permitted along much of the trail (although it is prohibited by state law on Sundays in both Connecticut and Massachusetts). Wear blaze orange from mid-October and late December, the most popular hunting season.

• Respect the private property along the trail.

• Be careful not to block trailhead gates when parking since work crews and emergency vehicles need access.

• Motorized vehicles are prohibited from the trail but off-road motorcycles and ATV's appear to still use it.

• The trail is open from sunrise to sunset.

ORIENTATION:

This description covers the far northern section of the Airline State Park Trail in Thompson, CT and the adjoining Southern New England Trunkline Tr. from Douglas to Franklin, MA. Other portions of the Airline State Park Trail are detailed in chapters 31 and 32.

This section of the trail currently exists in 3 parts and the surface varies considerably. The 17-mile leg from Rte. 200 in Thompson, CT to Rte. 146 in Uxbridge, MA offers the easiest and most scenic riding, especially in the area of Douglas State Forest where the trail's processed stone surface explores natural surroundings of open wetlands and shady forest. The 2.3 miles of trail between Rte. 146 and the

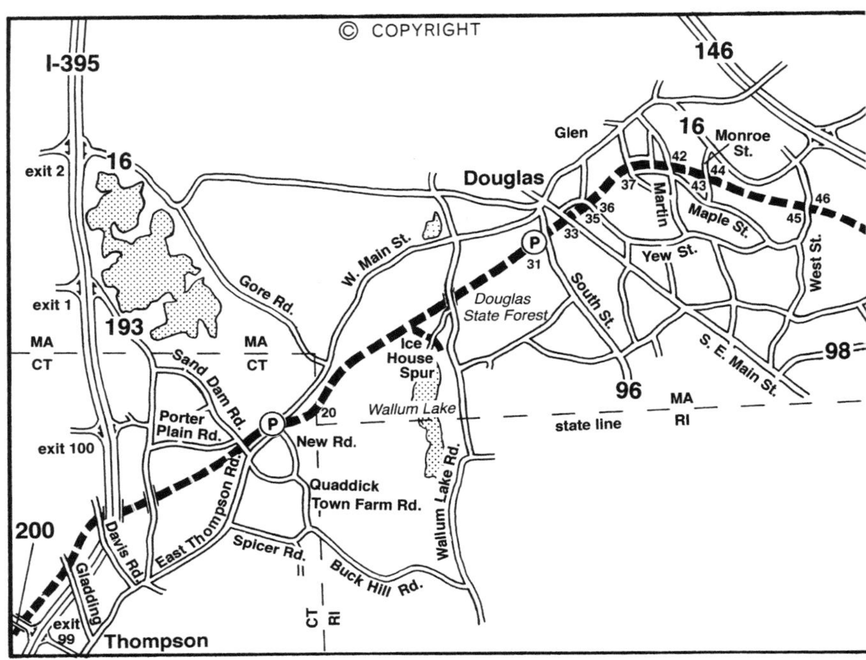

Blackstone River in Millville, MA are rideable but include an overgrown section. The 6.1 miles from the Blackstone River in Blackstone to Grove St. in Franklin, MA hold difficult conditions with rough and overgrown surfaces. On-road detours from the rail line are required to link these three parts.

Mountain bikes are advised. Much of the surface is either loose, rough, wet, or bermed with the up-and-down "washboard" effect of motorized usage. Missing bridges at many road intersections require negotiating steep slopes.

The trail's lowest points of elevation are the western terminus in Thompson, CT and the Blackstone River in Blackstone, MA. The highest points are Wallum Lake Rd. in Douglas, MA and the eastern terminus in Franklin, MA.

Parking is limited to gravel turnouts at a few road intersections, the largest and most popular being Rte. 96 in Douglas. Gates at road intersections along the western part of the trail in Massachusetts are numbered and displayed on the map to assist with tracking location. Note that well-used,

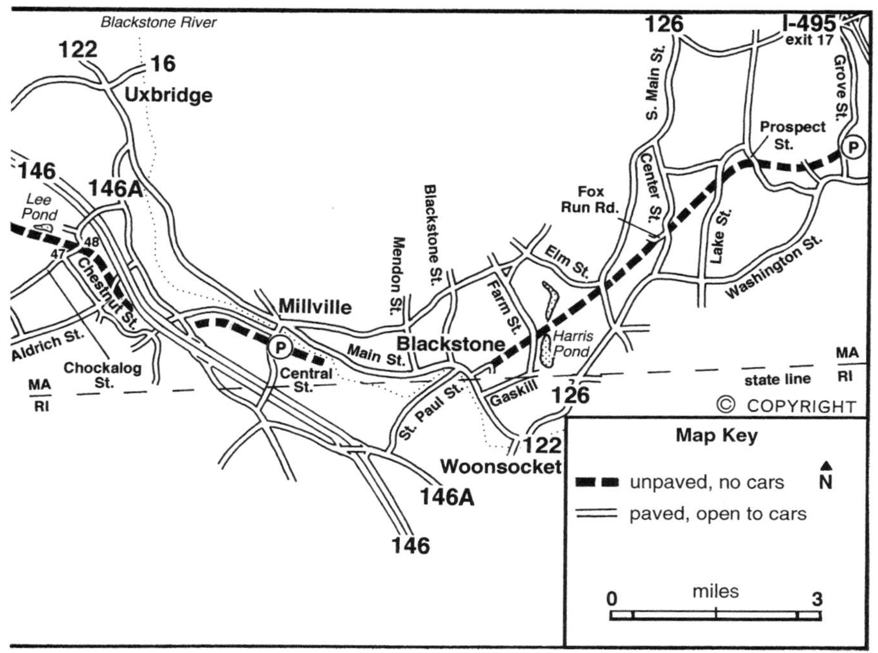

unmarked private paths intersect along the way so focus on the rail-trail's steady line and even grade when navigating.

TRAIL DESCRIPTION:

Begin in Thompson, CT at **East Thompson Rd.** Heading southwest, the **Airline State Park Trail** offers about 5 miles of challenging riding. The trip starts with a short climb up a scrabbly slope, continues over a gravelly area bermed from motorcycles, then narrows in woods with a smoother surface to **Sand Dam Rd.** The next mile and a half are straight and flat but more berms slow the pedaling.

The trail passes under **Rte. 193** (2.1 miles) and **I-395** (2.7 miles) and then remains within earshot of the highway for its remaining distance. It tilts uphill for most of the next mile, detouring where fill used for **Gladding Rd.** blocks the rail bed, and descends as it passes under **Rte. 200** (4.6 miles). The trail ends within another half-mile, becoming impassible due to erosion and poor drainage.

Smoother riding prevails northeast of East Thompson

Rd. The Airline contends with areas of berms and loose sand for a short distance to the Massachusetts **state line** at **gate 20** where it enters Douglas, MA as the **Southern New England Trunk Line Tr.** and gains a smoother surface.

A half-mile uphill slope beside Rocky Brook leads to several miles of enjoyable scenery along a string of open wetlands and small ponds in 5,000-acre **Douglas State Forest**. About 2.2 miles from East Thompson Rd. look for the **Ice House Spur Line** branching right (southeast) to the access road for the swimming beach at **Wallum Lake**.

Continuing on the main line, the trail reaches its highest elevation as it passes under a stone arch bridge carrying **Wallum Lake Rd.** (3.0 miles). It gains a slight downslope at this point and passes Morse Pond before reaching the **Rte. 96** trailhead at **gates 31/32** (4.6 miles).

The improved surface conditions extend eastward for a few more miles although horse hoof prints make some parts bumpy. The trail passes several homes and roads at the outskirts of Douglas and E. Douglas, then regains a woodsy feel after **Martin St.** (6.7 miles). It contends with berms on the way to **Monroe St.** (7.3 miles), enters Uxbridge, then drops abruptly to **West St.** (8.7 miles) at the site of a missing bridge. After passing **Lee Pond**, the trail intersects **Chockalog St.** at **gates 47/48** (10.5 miles), climbs a bank to cross **Aldrich St.** (**Rte. 98**) (11.2 miles), then dead ends at the four lanes of **Rte. 146** (12.1 miles).

Detour on roads to reach the next section. Returning to Aldrich St., turn right (east) and ride for a half-mile, turn right on **Rte. 146A** and ride for 1.2 miles, then look for the trail on the left at the top of a gravel slope. This 2.3-mile mid-section starts with berms and overgrown conditions until **Central St.** in **Millville**, where a smooth and firm surface extends to a decrepit bridge over the **Blackstone River**.

Detouring again, return to Central St. and turn right, turn right on **Rte. 122**, and ride for 2.9 miles. In **Blackstone**, turn left at the *Castle Hill* sign and follow the drive to a right-hand turn where the trail continues straight into woods.

This 6.1-mile section begins with overgrown conditions near the Rhode Island border, with the mills of Woonsocket visible across **Harris Pond** a mile ahead on the right. In Bellingham, the trail passes under **Rte. 126** and encounters a mile of drainage problems to **Fox Run Rd.** at the crossing of **Center St.**, and drops on a slope in order to cross **Lake St.** In Franklin, it diverts from the railbed to cross **Prospect St.** where a former bridge was filled, then contends with overgrowing branches and berms left from motorcycles for most of the remaining distance to **Grove St.**

BACKGROUND:

The Blackstone-Franklin, MA portion of this route originated in 1849 as part of the Norfolk County Railroad, and other portions were completed as part of the Boston & New York Central. The line grew through Connecticut as the Air Line Railroad which opened a direct route between Boston and New York City in 1873.

A 1955 flood destroyed the railroad's bridge over the Quinebaug River in Putnam, CT and a 1968 flood destroyed the bridge over the Blackstone River in Blackstone, MA, ending through service. Several years later, Connecticut and Massachusetts each acquired sections of the route for use as a recreational trail.

DRIVING DIRECTIONS:

East Thompson Rd., Thompson, CT: From I-395 take Exit 99 and follow Rte. 200 east to Thompson center. Turn left on Rte. 193 north and drive for 1.5 miles, then fork right on East Thompson Rd. After 2.5 miles, fork right at Sand Dam Rd., continue on East Thompson Rd. for 0.6 miles, then look for an unmarked gravel turnout at an S-turn.

Rte. 96, Douglas, MA: From I-395 take Exit 2 and follow Rte. 16 east for 6.8 miles, then turn right and follow Rte. 96 south for a half-mile to the trailhead, on the right.

Grove St., Franklin, MA: From I-495 take Exit 17 and follow Rte. 140 north for 0.1 miles, then turn left on Grove St. and continue for 2.1 miles. Park beside the road on the left where the rail-trail intersects.

TOILETS:

Douglas State Forest on Wallum Lake Rd. (in season)

ADDITIONAL INFORMATION:

Douglas State Forest, (508) 476-7872

34 Thompson Heritage Way

Thompson, CT

LENGTH: 1.5 miles
SURFACE: mostly paved, some stone dust
TERRAIN: mostly flat

Thompson Heritage Way ties two local parks together with a short ride past an 1800's mill village.

RULES & SAFETY:

• Bicyclists should yield to pedestrians.

• Be extra cautious when children and pets are present since their movements can be unpredictable.

• Keep to the right, pass on the left, and alert others (*"On your left..."*) when approaching from behind.

• At Heritage Way Park, swimming is not permitted in the pond and glass containers are forbidden.

• Dogs must be leashed and their wastes removed.

• The area is open from dawn to dusk.

ORIENTATION:

In general, the southern portion of the trail lies in a more developed area of the village and the northern portion explores a wooded area. The trail intersects four roads along its midsection with crosswalks in place at each. Trailheads include Riverside Park which has easy access and also serves a baseball field, the library which provides toilet facilities when it's open, and Heritage Way Park which offers picnic tables and also serves as a boat launch.

TRAIL DESCRIPTION:

Begin at **Riverside Park** where a gazebo and lawn greet visitors along a narrow space beside the **French River**. From the park entrance on **Main St.**, the **Heritage Way** path follows the riverbank upstream past a baseball field and rises on a pedestrian bridge spanning the river. Turning right on the other side, it follows the edge of the parking lot for the **Thompson Library and Community**

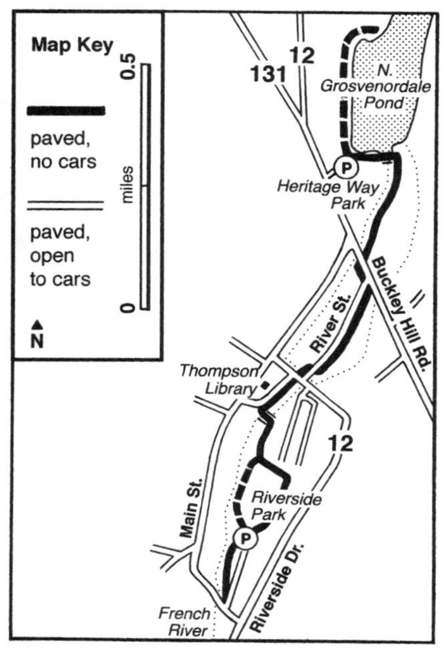

Center and joins a sidewalk for a short distance to **Rte. 12**, where it intersects at a crosswalk. The trail follows a short boardwalk to the intersection of **River St.** and continues north between its wooden guardrail and the river, passing the village's vast mill building on the left.

Reaching **Buckley Hill Rd.** at the end, the trail turns left beside the street, climbs a short slope, then crosses and continues into woods along a canal which provided water power for the mill. Curving upstream, the trail and canal emerge at **N. Grosvenordale Pond** with a view of its dam and spillway, then turn left (west) along the southern shore.

Just ahead, the trail passes a parking lot, picnic tables, and another water view at **Heritage Way Park**, then returns to woods on a stone dust surface which extends for a quarter-mile up the western shore.

DRIVING DIRECTIONS:

I-395 northbound: Take Exit 98 and join Rte. 12 north for 2 miles. Turn left on Main St., then immediately right at the park entrance.

I-395 southbound: Take Exit 99 and follow Rte. 200 west for 1 mile. Turn right on Rte. 12 north and drive for 1 mile, turn left on Main St., then immediately right at the park entrance.

TOILETS:

at the library, when it's open

ADDITIONAL INFORMATION:

Town of Thompson Community Dev., (860) 923-9475

35 Quinebaug River Trail

Killingly, CT

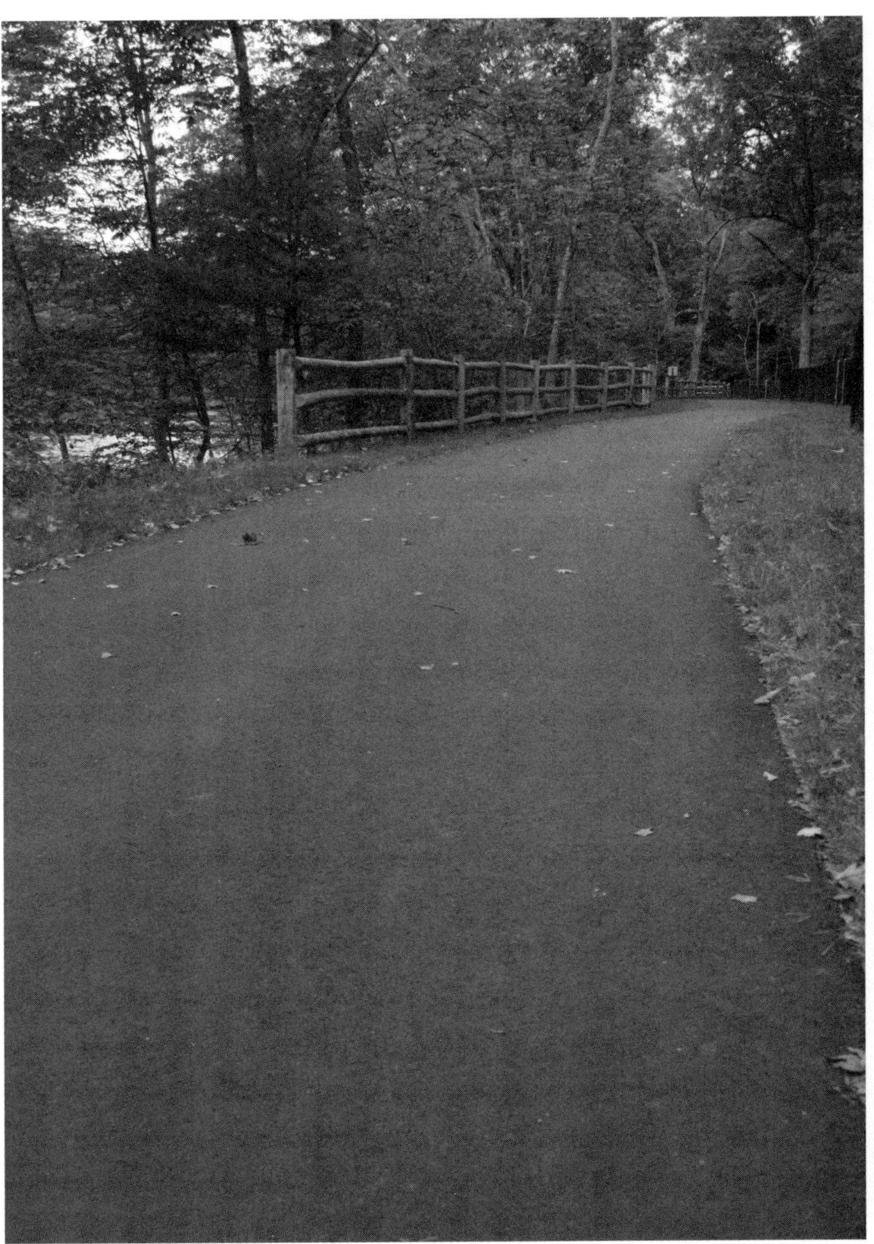

LENGTH: 2.9 miles
SURFACE: paved
TERRAIN: small slopes

Following an old trolley line for part of the way, this recreation path connects the village of Danielson with peaceful scenery along the Quinebaug River.

RULES & SAFETY:

- Bicyclists should yield to pedestrians.
- Keep to the right, pass on the left, and alert others (*"On your left..."*) when approaching from behind.
- Ride at a safe speed, and use extra caution when children and pets are present.
- Respect the private property along the trail.
- Help keep it clean by carrying out all that you carry in.
- The trail is open only during daylight hours.

ORIENTATION:

The trail has a north-south alignment and follows the Quinebaug River for its entire length. It begins with a crosswalk at a busy intersection and a separated pathway paralleling Rte. 6/Rte. 12, reduces to a sidewalk for a short distance along Rte. 12, then turns away from the roadway and enjoys much quieter, more natural surroundings while passing a few dead end residential streets.

Trailhead access is available at the northern terminus in Danielson (which involves using a crosswalk at Rte. 6/ Rte. 12) and at a complex of baseball fields off Rte. 12.

TRAIL DESCRIPTION:

From the Water St. trailhead parking lot, follow the crosswalk across **Rte. 6/Rte. 12** to reach the trail at Overlook 2. Turning to the right, it runs for only a short distance to Overlook 1, built above the confluence of the **Quinebaug River** and **Five Mile River**.

Turning to the left, the trail follows a strip of parkland between the river and the road and passes two more overlooks in an area of plantings, benches, and picnic tables. At Overlook 4 it merges with the edge of Rte. 12 and

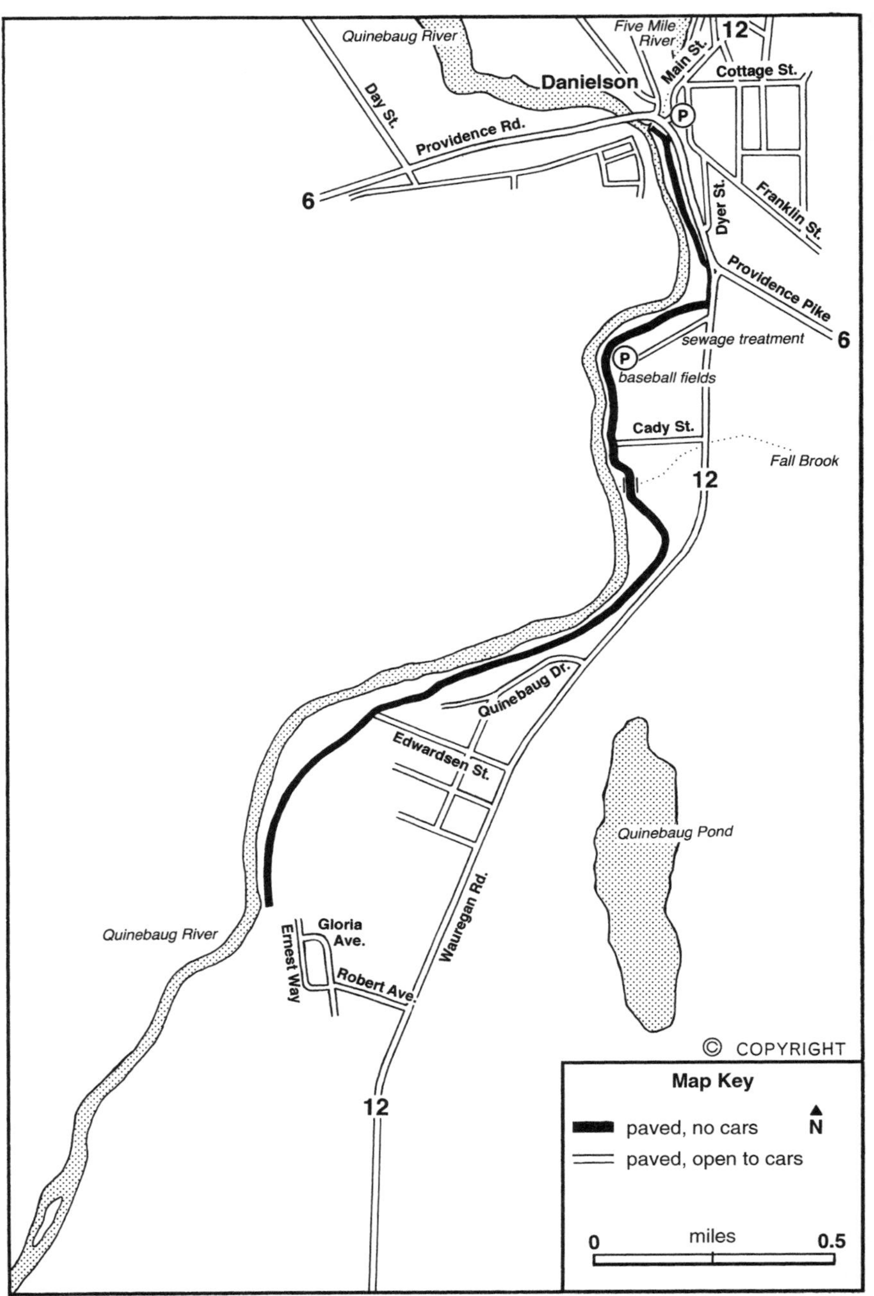
Quinebaug River
Five Mile River
12
Main St.
Cottage St.
Danielson
Day St.
Providence Rd.
P
6
Dyer St.
Franklin St.
Providence Pike
sewage treatment
6
P
baseball fields
Cady St.
Fall Brook
12
Quinebaug Dr.
Edwardsen St.
Quinebaug Pond
Wauregan Rd.
Gloria Ave.
Ernest Way
Robert Ave.
Quinebaug River
12
© COPYRIGHT
Map Key
paved, no cars
paved, open to cars
N
0
miles
0.5

follows a short section of sidewalk, then turns sharply right just before a **sewage treatment plant**.

A sign marks the next section of trail as it heads west, descending a slight slope to the side of the river and then circling a complex of **baseball fields**. A parking lot here serves as an alternate trailhead. Bending back to the south, it enters the shade of woods and curves through trees with views over the water for most of the next half-mile.

The trail passes the end of **Cady St.** at the 1.1-mile mark where it turns away from the riverbank and crosses a bridge over **Fall Brook**. It then joins the bed of an old trolley line for the remaining distance, beginning on a gentle uphill grade along the base of a slope below Rte. 12 with the river visible through woods on the right.

The trail crests this hill near **Quinebaug Dr.** (2.1 miles) and descends beside a small clearing to the end of **Edwardsen St.** (2.3 miles). It straightens in flat terrain and the shade of forest for the remaining half-mile before dead-ending in woods beside the river.

BACKGROUND:

The Quinebaug River Trail's origin lies with a state highway reconstruction project in Danielson. When the rotary intersection of Rte. 6 and Rte. 12 was reconfigured with a traffic signal in 1991, extra space along the Quinebaug River was utilized for a park and pathway. The path doubled in length in 1995 when it was extended through town-owned lands, then was extended again along a former trolley line ten years later. With more progress, the trail will continue southward to the Plainfield town line.

DRIVING DIRECTIONS:

From I-395 take Exit 91W and follow Rte. 6 west to its junction with Rte. 12. Continue on Rte. 6 west/Rte. 12 north for a short distance to the next intersection, where the two split. Turn right on Rte. 12 north, then immediately right on Water St. and park in the lot on the right marked by a *"River Trail Parking"* sign.

TOILETS:

none are provided

ADDITIONAL INFORMATION:

Planning & Development, Town of Killingly, Tel. (860) 779-5311

36 Bluff Point State Park

Groton, CT

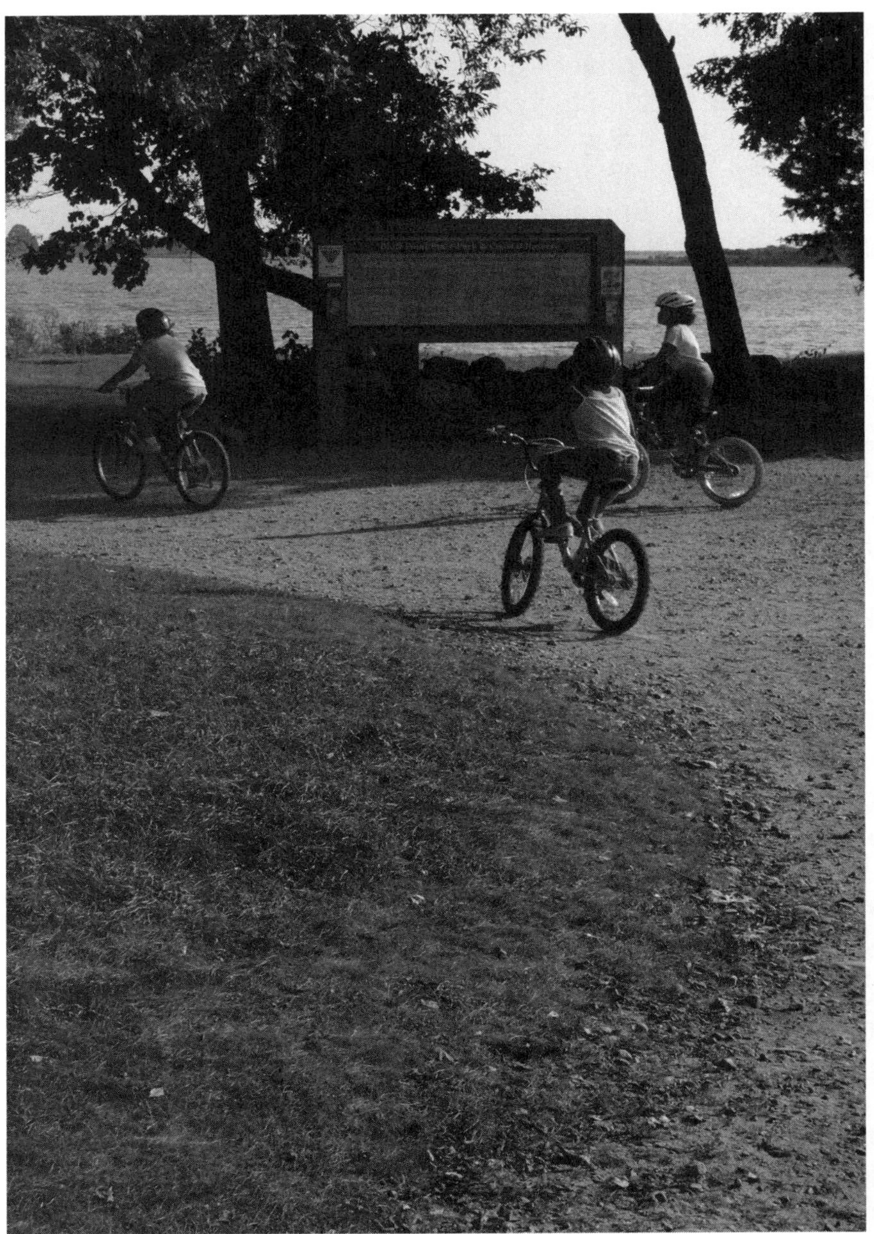

LENGTH: 5 miles
SURFACE: mostly gravel, some paved
TERRAIN: small hills

Together with nearby Haley Farm State Park, Bluff Point offers smooth trails for biking and pretty coastal scenery. Bring your bathing suit and a picnic.

RULES & SAFETY:

- Bicyclists should yield to pedestrians.
- Keep to the right, pass on the left, and alert others (*"On your left..."*) when approaching from behind.
- Ride at a safe speed and use extra caution when children and pets are present.
- Stay on the trail surface to minimize impacts.
- Dogs must be leashed and their wastes removed.
- The park is open during daylight hours.

ORIENTATION:

Both Bluff Point and Haley Farm are trailheads, but Bluff Point's also serves a beach (at the end of the peninsula) which can be crowded in summer. Trail signs are few but the shoreline, a railroad, and surrounding streets provide helpful landmarks. Only the smoothest trails are shown on the map; many other rougher paths intersect along the way.

TRAIL DESCRIPTION:

Starting from the **Bluff Point State Park** trailhead, the most popular trail runs south along the **Poquonnock River** to the beach at the end of the peninsula. Continue past the trailhead signs on its broad, gravel surface and keep right at the first intersection. Rolling with a few small hills in woods along the shore, it passes a second intersection after a mile, rises on a final slope at the 1.4-mile mark, and descends the other side to the **beach** access point (1.5 miles).

Just ahead, the trail tops a small knoll for a view of **Long Island Sound** before looping back to the north on a hillier, rougher 1.2-mile route which is best suited for wide-tired bikes. After climbing to the peninsula's highest

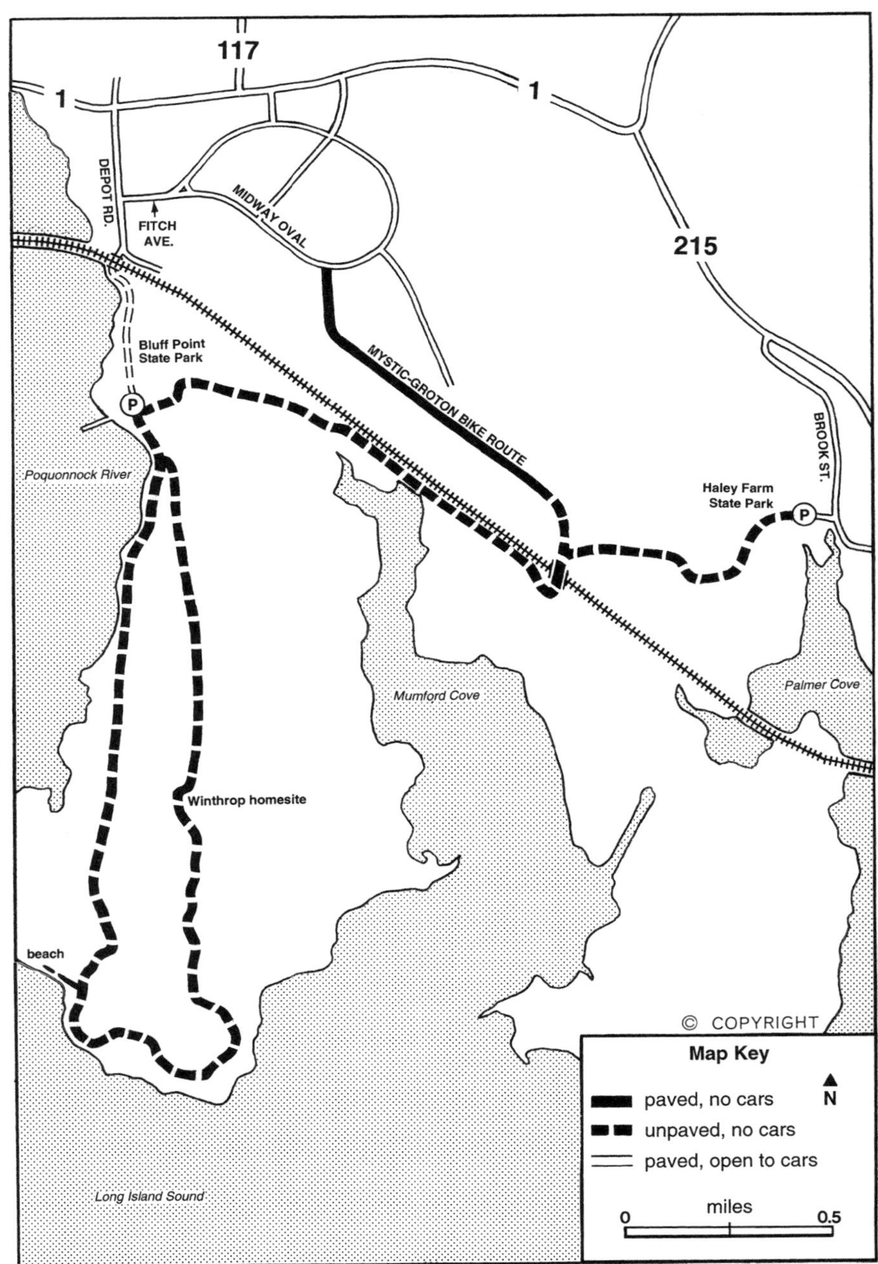
117
1
1
215
DEPOT RD.
FITCH AVE.
MIDWAY OVAL
MYSTIC-GROTON BIKE ROUTE
Bluff Point State Park
P
Poquonnock River
Haley Farm State Park
P
BROOK ST.
Mumford Cove
Palmer Cove
Winthrop homesite
beach
Long Island Sound
© COPYRIGHT
Map Key
paved, no cars
unpaved, no cars
paved, open to cars
N
miles
0
0.5

elevation at the **Winthrop homesite** it descends for 0.8 miles back to the trailhead with a few rough spots.

The trail running eastward to **Haley Farm State Park** is smooth and flat. It merges beside railroad tracks at a view of **Mumford Cove** after a half-mile, climbs a slope and crosses a bridge over the tracks (1 mile), and soon intersects the **Mystic-Groton Bike Route**, marked by a sign.

Turning right, this bike route curves through woods on a gentle downslope to the large stone walls and old fields of Haley Farm. Turning left, the route follows a utility corridor to **Midway Oval** with surfaces of gravel and old pavement. Return to the Bluff Point trailhead by turning left on **Midway Oval**, left on **Fitch Ave.**, and left on **Depot St.**, then keep right at the park entrance which dips underneath the railroad.

BACKGROUND:

Bluff Point became a popular vacation destination in the 1920's and hosted an amusement park, campground, and close to 100 summer cottages until a hurricane destroyed much of the area in 1938. As nature reclaimed the land, the state began acquiring portions of the peninsula in 1963 and the park now totals 806 acres.

The nearby Haley Farm State Park property has a long history of owners, including Connecticut's first governor, John Winthrop. From 1869 until 1924, Caleb Henry farmed the land and created its immense stone walls using a so-called stone-puller, a unique device drawn by oxen and able to manipulate 3-ton boulders. Threatened by development proposals in the 1960's, the land was saved by a local fundraising effort which established the 198-acre park in 1970.

DRIVING DIRECTIONS:

Bluff Point State Park: From I-95 take Exit 88 and follow Rte. 117 south. Turn right on Rte. 1 west for 0.2 miles, turn left on Depot Rd., then bear right at the park entrance (passing under the railroad). Park in the lot at the end.

Haley Farm State Park: From I-95 take Exit 88 and follow Rte. 117 south. Turn left on Rte. 1 east for 0.9 miles, turn right (south) on Rte. 215 for a half-mile, then turn right on Brook St. for a half-mile. Turn right on Haley Farm La. and park in the lot at the end.

TOILETS:

Bluff Point State Park trailhead, Haley Farm State Park trailhead

37 Washington Secondary Bike Path Moosup Valley State Park Trail

Cranston, RI - Plainfield, CT

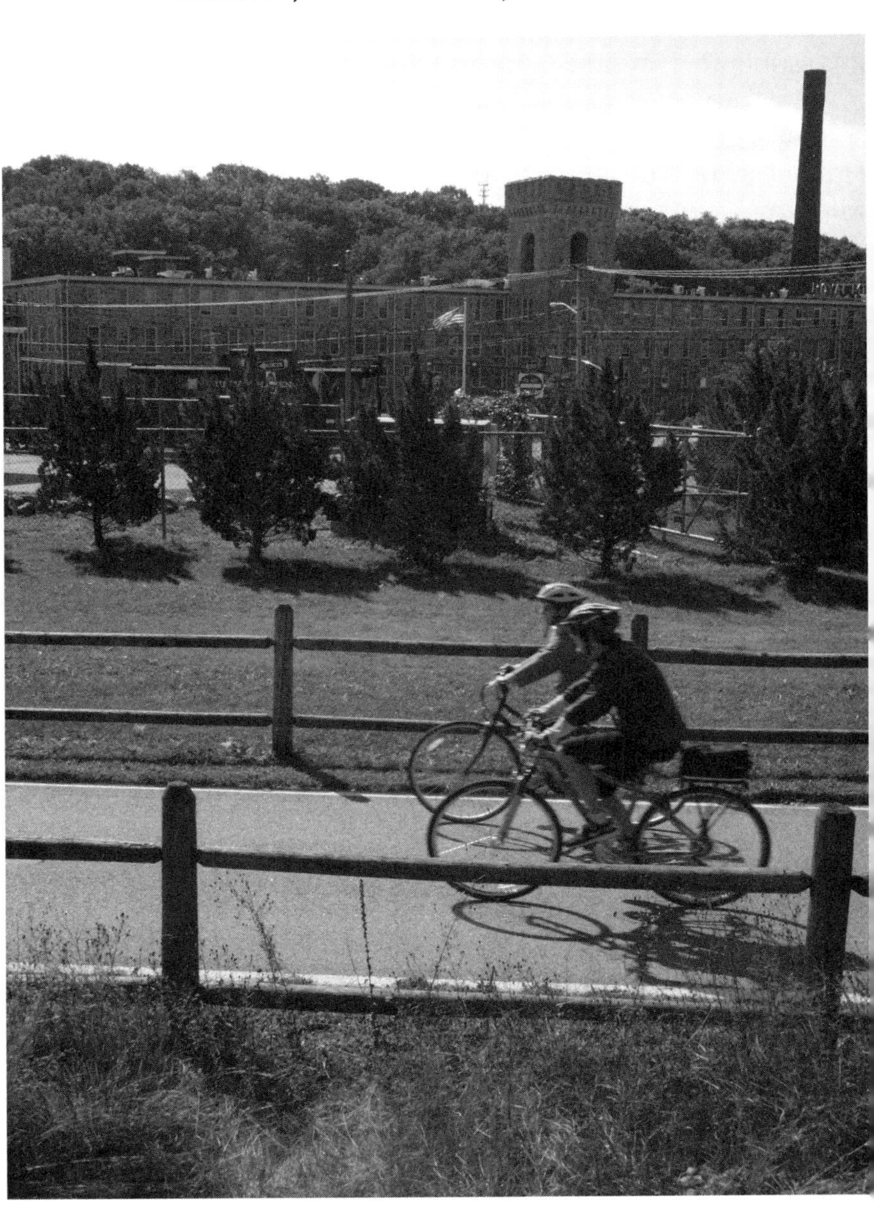

LENGTH: 30.6 miles
SURFACE: half the trail is paved, half is unpaved and rough
TERRAIN: gentle slopes
NOTE: mountain bikes recommended for unpaved sections

The area's longest rail-trail stretches from the edge of Providence to rural woodlands in eastern Connecticut with a great variety of scenes along the way. The paved sections allow easy rolling but the unpaved ones hold challenging conditions.

RULES & SAFETY:

• Bicyclists should yield to pedestrians.

• Keep to the right, pass on the left, and alert others (*"On your left..."*) when approaching from behind.

• Note that walkers are requested to use the left side in Rhode Island.

• Ride at a safe speed, and use extra caution when children and pets are present since their movements can be unpredictable.

• Respect the private property along the trail, and carry out all that you carry in.

• Parts of the trail are remote so be self-sufficient with water, food, and bike repair supplies.

• Hunting is permitted along the western half of the trail, so wear blaze orange clothing in late fall, the most popular hunting season.

• Motorized uses are prohibited but appear to make use of the trail's undeveloped western sections.

• Dogs must be leashed and their wastes removed.

• The trail is open from sunrise to sunset.

ORIENTATION:

In Rhode Island, this rail-trail is known as the Washington Secondary Bike Path which consists of several local trails called the Cranston Bike Path, Warwick Greenway, West Warwick Greenway, Coventry Greenway, and the Trestle Trail. In Connecticut, the route is known as the Moosup Valley State Park Trail.

The trail spans a long distance and encounters an especially wide range of conditions and surroundings, so plan your ride accordingly. The paved, eastern half in Rhode Island gets the most usage and runs through commercial and residential areas in Cranston and Warwick, then past mill villages and river scenery in West Warwick and Coventry. The western half explores rural woodlands from Coventry, RI to Plainfield, CT and has mostly undeveloped conditions with difficult biking and relatively little usage.

The trail's highest elevation is the settlement of Summit in western Rhode Island and its lowest elevations are the Pawtuxet River bridge near I-295 in Warwick, RI and the western terminus at Moosup, CT. Trailhead parking lots are available at numerous points in Rhode Island but only roadside parking exists along the trail in Connecticut.

TRAIL DESCRIPTION:

Begin at the Cranston, RI end where the trail is known locally as the **Cranston Bike Path**. Accessed from the edge

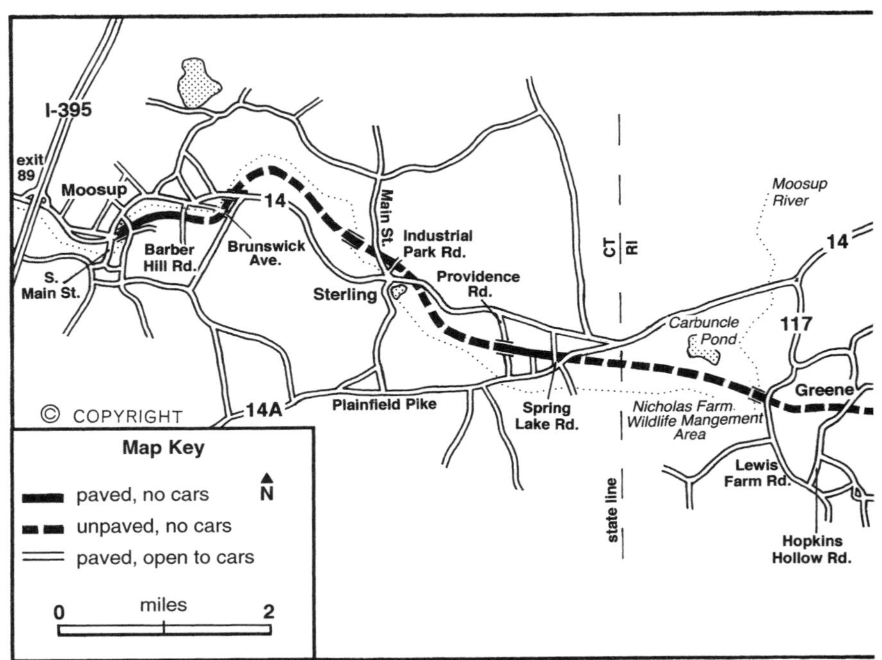

of a Lowe's parking lot on **Garfield Ave.**, the trail heads to the right (north) for only a quarter-mile and intersects a short side loop around neighboring Tongue Pond along the way. Heading left (south), 14.2 miles of paved trail continue past the back of the Lowes store and into the shade of a tree-covered corridor. Beginning in a mix of commercial and residential areas, riders pass under **Gansett Ave.** at the 0.8-mile mark but should use caution ahead when crossing at **Dyer Ave.** and busy **Rte. 12** (**Park Ave.**) (1.4 miles) where a crosswalk signal proves useful.

The surroundings get a bit leafier as the bike path passes under **Rte. 5** (2.0 miles) in an area of residential neighborhoods but the trail eventually returns to a commercial area along Oaklawn Ave. (Rte. 5) for three quarters of a mile after the underpass for **Rte. 37** (3.5 miles). The next mile holds more natural scenery with a bridge crossing Meshanticut Brook near the 5-mile mark and under-passes allowing easy rolling past surrounding roads.

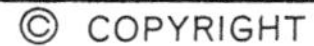

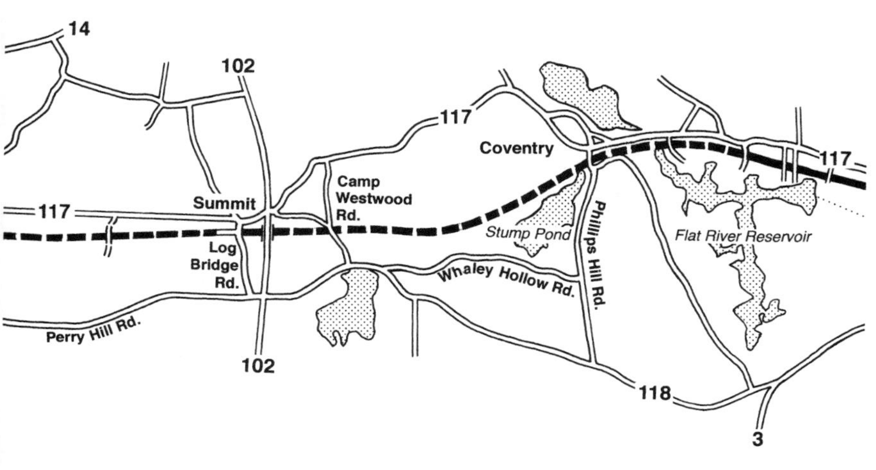

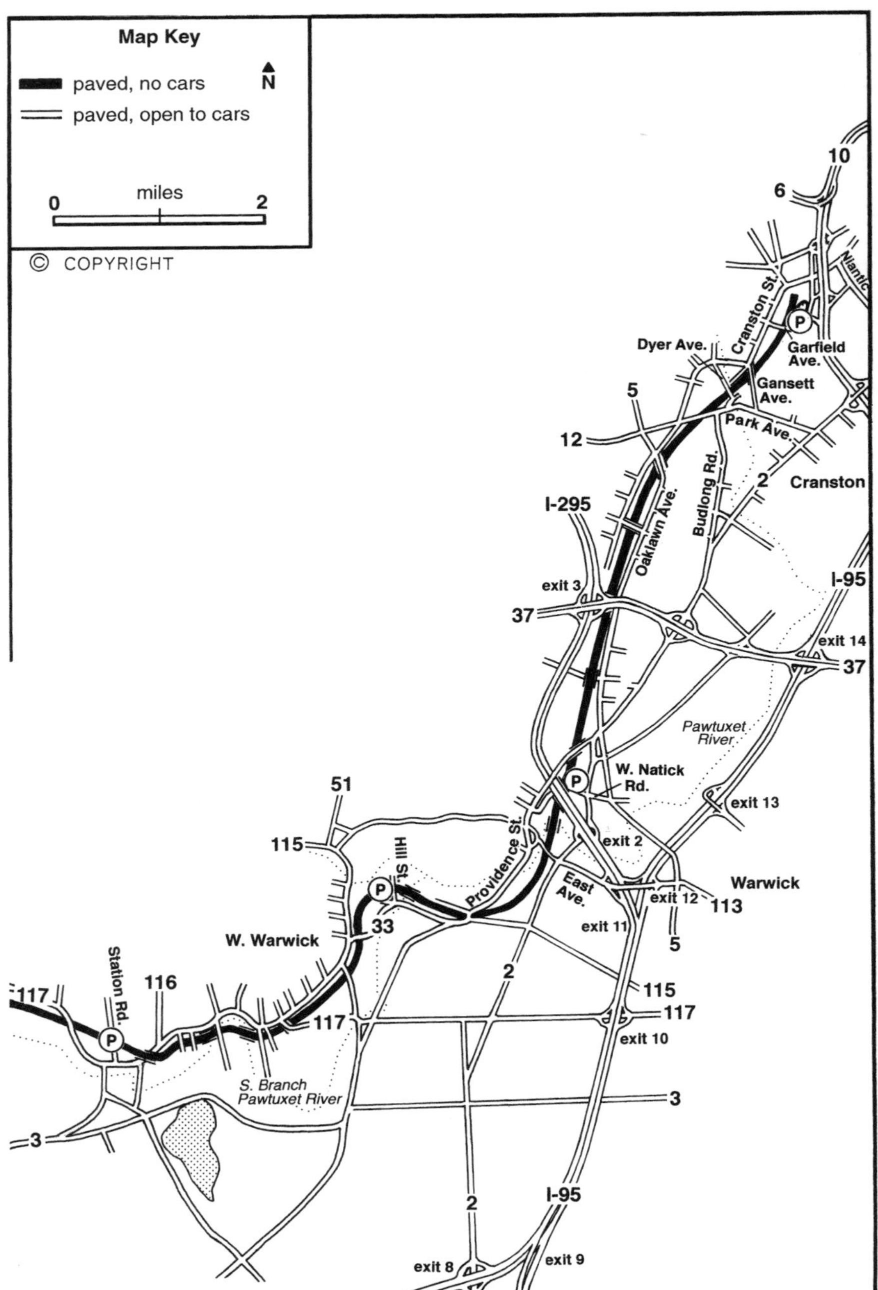

Map Key
paved, no cars
paved, open to cars
N
miles
0
2
© COPYRIGHT
10
6
Niantic
Cranston St.
P
Garfield Ave.
Dyer Ave.
Gansett Ave.
5
Park Ave.
12
Budlong Rd.
Oaklawn Ave.
2
Cranston
I-295
I-95
exit 3
37
exit 14
37
Pawtuxet River
P
W. Natick Rd.
51
exit 13
115
Hill St.
Providence St.
exit 2
P
East Ave.
Warwick
exit 12
113
33
exit 11
W. Warwick
5
Station Rd.
116
2
115
117
117
117
P
exit 10
S. Branch Pawtuxet River
3
3
2
I-95
exit 8
exit 9

The bike path enters Warwick as the **Warwick Greenway** just before the trailhead parking area at **West Natick Rd.** where the two bridges of **I-295** (5.5 miles) create noise overhead. Peace and quiet soon return and the trail crosses a large bridge over the **Pawtuxet River** (5.7 miles), then intersects busy **East Ave.** (6.1 miles) where it tilts upward on a noticeable slope and begins a long righthand bend to the west.

The trail straightens and enters West Warwick at the intersection of **Rte. 33** (**Providence St.**) (7.2 miles) where crosswalk signals help it through the traffic and a sign marks the start of the **West Warwick Greenway**. It crosses a bridge over both the **South Branch Pawtuxet River** (7.8 miles) and the stone buildings of an 1800's mill complex, and passes a trailhead parking lot on **Hill St.** Arcing southward with a lefthand curve, the trail reaches a second crossing of Rte. 33 (Providence St.) at the village of **Arctic** (8.7 miles) and gets a view of another huge stone mill building.

The trail follows the river for a short distance and rises on another uphill slope for the next few miles as it slowly turns back to the west. It slips under a bridge carrying **Rte. 117** (9.9 miles) at the Coventry town line to become the **Coventry Greenway**, intersects three roads as it passes an industrial complex, then crosses a second bridge over the South Branch (10.3 miles) with a nice view over the water. Just ahead, it passes another mill, crosses a third bridge over the river (10.7 miles), and crosses a bridge over Rte. 117 (11.2 miles) as it flattens at the village of **Washington**. Just ahead, the trail crosses **Station Rd.** (11.6 miles) at a popular trailhead parking lot.

To the west, the pavement lasts for another 2.4 miles. The bike path passes town recreation fields, intersects Rte. 117, and continues into woodsy suroundings intersperced with a few industrial locations. It reaches a view of **Flat River Reservoir** (13.3 miles) on the left and, aside from crossing a few deserted roads, enjoys purely natural scenery along its northern shore.

The pavement currently ends at the 14.2-mile mark where the rougher **Trestle Trail** begins. In places, its gravel surface has a wave-like pattern of berms left from motorized usage in addition to a few detours at missing bridges and areas of poor drainage. This is proven a short distance ahead where the trail returns to the reservoir's shoreline and is halted by a missing bridge over a narrow channel (15.1 miles). To continue, riders must dismount and use steep footpaths on both sides of the water linking the bridge for parallel Rte. 117.

The trail narrows and begins another uphill slope at this point as encroaching tree limbs and less usage give it a more remote feel. After crossing **Phillips Hill Rd.** (15.5 miles), it crosses a bridge at the outlet of **Stump Pond** where a pretty water view spreads to the south. Note that this bridge lacks railings, so use caution.

Climbing at a slight pace, the trail is surrounded by woods for the next few miles. It contends with a missing bridge at Quidnick Brook (17.1 miles) where a detour foot-path could create wet feet, then scrambles up a steep banking at **Camp Westwood Rd.** (18.2 miles) where a former bridge over the railroad has been filled. Just ahead, drainage problems mire the trail as it passes under a bridge for **Rte. 102** (18.8 miles) with vast puddles spanning the entire width of the railbed.

The uphill grade ends at this point and the trail reaches its highest elevation at the crossing of **Log Bridge Rd.** (19.1 miles) and the settlement of **Summit**. It continues westward on a paved dead end road before returning to woods where it borders scenic wetlands along the next two miles with difficult pedaling due to motorcycle berms and another area of poor drainage. A missing bridge over Bucks Horn Brook requires the fording of another stream just before the cluster of houses at **Greene** on **Hopkins Hollow Rd.** (21.7 miles).

A crushed stone surface, loose in places, leads the trail down a slight slope between stone walls to **Lewis Farm**

Rd. (22.5 miles). The trail crosses a high, wooden bridge over the **Moosup River** (22.6 miles), which it follows downstream for the remaining miles, and enters the **Nicholas Farm Wildlife Management Area** which protects the next two miles of woodland scenery.

A wetland beside **Carbuncle Pond** opens the view on the right after a third of a mile and the surface becomes smoother as a scrub oak and pitch pine forest surrounds the trail near Riconn Airport, an air strip which is audible but not visible near the Rhode Island-Connecticut **state line** (24.5 miles).

Entering Sterling, CT, the trail emerges from woods at **Rte. 14A** (**Plainfield Pike**) (25.0 miles) and soon hits **Spring Lake Rd.** where the surface improves to asphalt for a half-mile near the village of Oneco. After a bike/pedestrian bridge carries the trail over **Providence Rd.** (25.6 miles), the surface reverts to gravel which has loose sand in places and more motorcycle berms. The trail passes through a cut in the bedrock of a small hillside where walls of blasted ledge line both sides, then curves to the right (northwest) and gains a smoother, firmer surface before intersecting **Rte. 14** (26.8 miles) near the center of **Sterling**.

The trail skirts a clearing, crosses **Industrial Park Rd.** and **Main St.** (27.2 miles), then returns to the shade of woods. In a short distance it crosses a second bridge over the Moosup River and continues along a straight line beside its course for the next mile, reaching the Plainfield town line along the way. A rollercoaster of small berms makes it a bumpy ride but several views of the river and its wetlands add scenic appeal.

Rounding the north side of Webb Hill, the trail bends left (southwest) on a half-mile-long curve, passes under a high bridge for Rte. 14 (29.0 miles), and intersects **Brunswick Ave.** near Glen Falls and an old textile mill site. It turns back to the west and intersects **Barber Hill Rd.** (29.7 miles) in another half-mile, where it gains an asphalt surface for the remaining 0.7 miles.

Following the open corridor of a utility line, the trail continues downstream, crosses River St., and reaches a final bridge over the flow at the village of **Moosup** where it ends at a commercial area off **S. Main St.**, 30.4 miles from the trailhead at Lowes in Cranston, RI.

BACKGROUND:

The Washington Secondary line was completed in 1854 by the Hartford, Providence, and Fishkill Railroad to link Connecticut, Rhode Island, and New York with freight and passenger service. As automobiles and trucks became popular in the 1900's, the railroad's importance began to fade and passenger service on this section of the line ended in 1930. Freight service lasted until 1988, and the tracks were removed a short time later.

Segments of the line were later sold to the states of Rhode Island and Connecticut and to the town of Coventry for recreational use. The rail-trail has been developed in stages, with Coventry's first 1.5 miles completed in 1998. Future improvements are planned for the western half of the trail where most of the rail bed remains undeveloped and, as a result, seldom used.

The Washington Secondary Bike Path and the Moosup Valley State Park Trail are designated as part of the East Coast Greenway, a planned multi-use trail from Maine to Florida.

DRIVING DIRECTIONS:

Garfield Ave., Cranston, RI: From I-95 take Exit 16 and follow Rte. 10 north. Take the Niantic Ave. exit, turn left at the end of the ramp on Niantic Ave., and continue to the next traffic signal. Turn left on Cranston St. and continue to the next traffic signal, turn left on Garfield Ave. and drive for a half-mile, then turn right at the large Lowes parking lot. Keep right and follow the perimeter of the parking lot to the rear corner of the building, where trail access and parking are provided.

West Natick Rd., Warwick, RI: From I-295 take Exit 2 and follow Rte. 2 north. Take the 2nd left on W. Natick Rd. and continue for a quarter-mile to the trailhead under the highway bridge.

Hay St., West Warwick, RI: From I-95, take Exit 10A if southbound or Exit 10 if northbound and follow Rte. 117 east for a short distance. Turn left on Rte. 115 west and drive for 2.9 miles, then turn right on Hay St. Turn immediately left at the caboose and find the parking lot ahead on the right, beside the trail.

Station Rd., Coventry, RI from points south on I-95: Take Exit 6 and follow Rte. 3 north for 3.7 miles. Turn left on Rte. 33 north and continue for a half-mile, then turn left on Rte. 117 west and continue for a quarter-mile. Turn right on Station Rd. and look for trailhead parking 0.2 miles ahead on both sides of the road.

Station Rd., Coventry, RI, from points north and east on I-95: Take Exit 10A if southbound or Exit 10 if northbound and follow Rte. 117 west for about 4.8 miles. Turn right on Station Rd. and find the trailhead 0.2 miles ahead on both sides of the road.

Main St., Moosup, CT: From I-395 take Exit 89 and follow Rte. 14 east for 1 mile to the stop sign in Moosup, where Rte. 14 turns left. The trail begins straight ahead at a large trestle bridge over Moosup River. Find designated roadside parking, and do not park in the private lot at the bridge.

TOILETS:

none on site

ADDITIONAL INFORMATION:

Connecticut Dept. of Environmental Protection, (860) 424-3200
Coventry Parks & Recreation, (401) 822-9107
Pawtuxet River Watershed Council, pawtuxet.org
Rhode Island Dept. of Environmental Management, (401) 222-6800

38 William C. O'Neill Bike Path

South Kingstown - Narragansett, RI

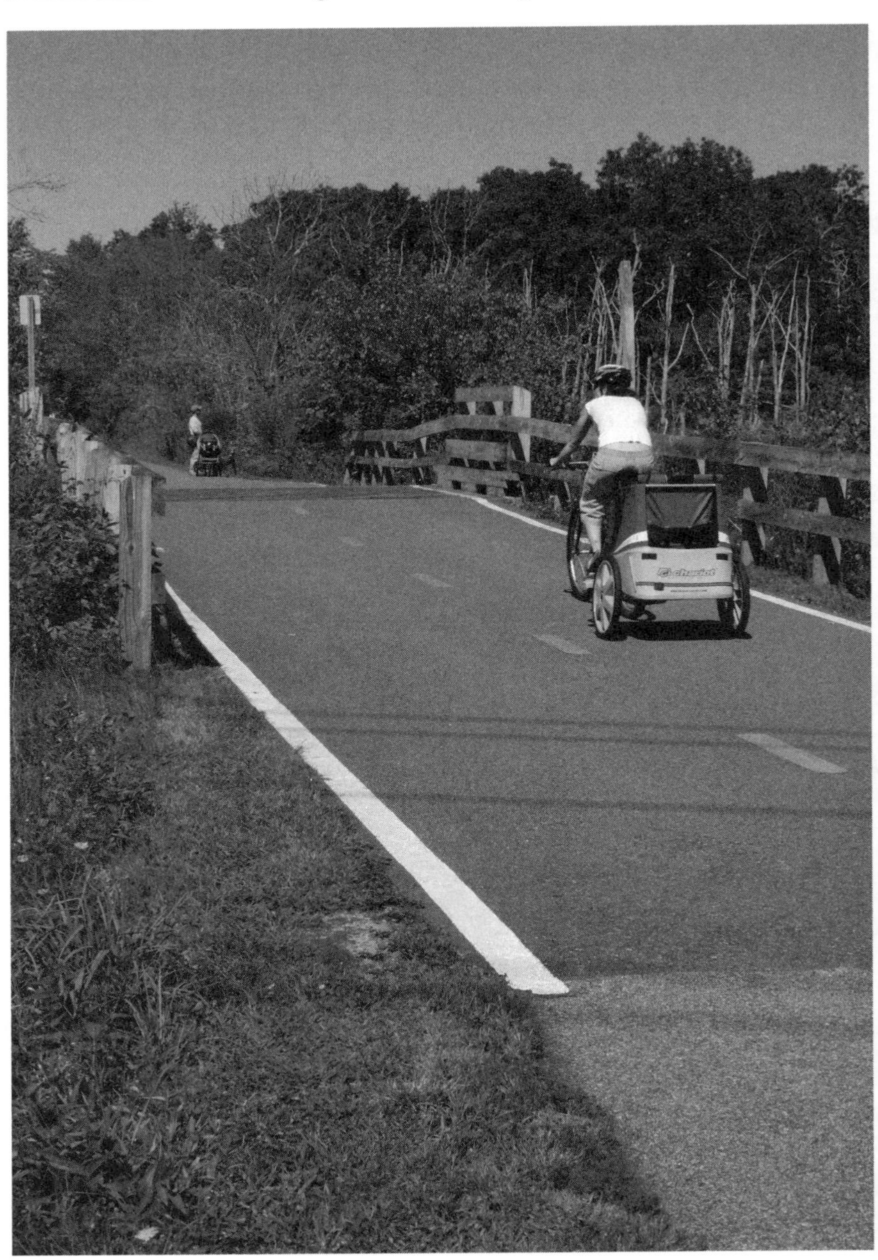

LENGTH: 7.2 miles, including (2) 0.2-mile on-road sections
SURFACE: paved
TERRAIN: gentle slopes

Also known as the South County Bike Path, this rail-trail is a car-free connection between a train station, schools, parks, village centers, and the seacoast. Miles of quiet scenery lie in between.

RULES & SAFETY:

- Bicyclists should yield to pedestrians.
- Keep to the right, pass on the left, and alert others (*"On your left..."*) when approaching from behind to avoid startling them.
- Note that walkers are asked to use the left side.
- Use extra caution when children and pets are present since their movements can be unpredictable.
- Help keep it clean by carrying out all that you carry in.
- Dogs must be leashed and their wastes removed.
- Bicycles and skateboards are not welcome in and around the Kingston Station building.
- The trail is open from dawn to dusk.

ORIENTATION:

The trail is well-developed with signs and crosswalks at road intersections, fencing along steep bankings, and benches and informational signs stationed at points of interest along the way. Mileage markers are posted along the trail and originate at Kingston Station, and street names are posted at many road crossings to assist visitors with determining their location.

The primary trailhead is Kingston Station at the western end of the trail. (Note that high speed trains occasionally pass the station and their sudden approach can be startling.) The western half of the trail holds the most natural scenery and the eastern half passes through residential areas and the village centers at Peace Dale and Wakefield. The trail has two 0.2-mile gaps along the eastern half where it follows quiet residential streets. A 1.2-mile on-

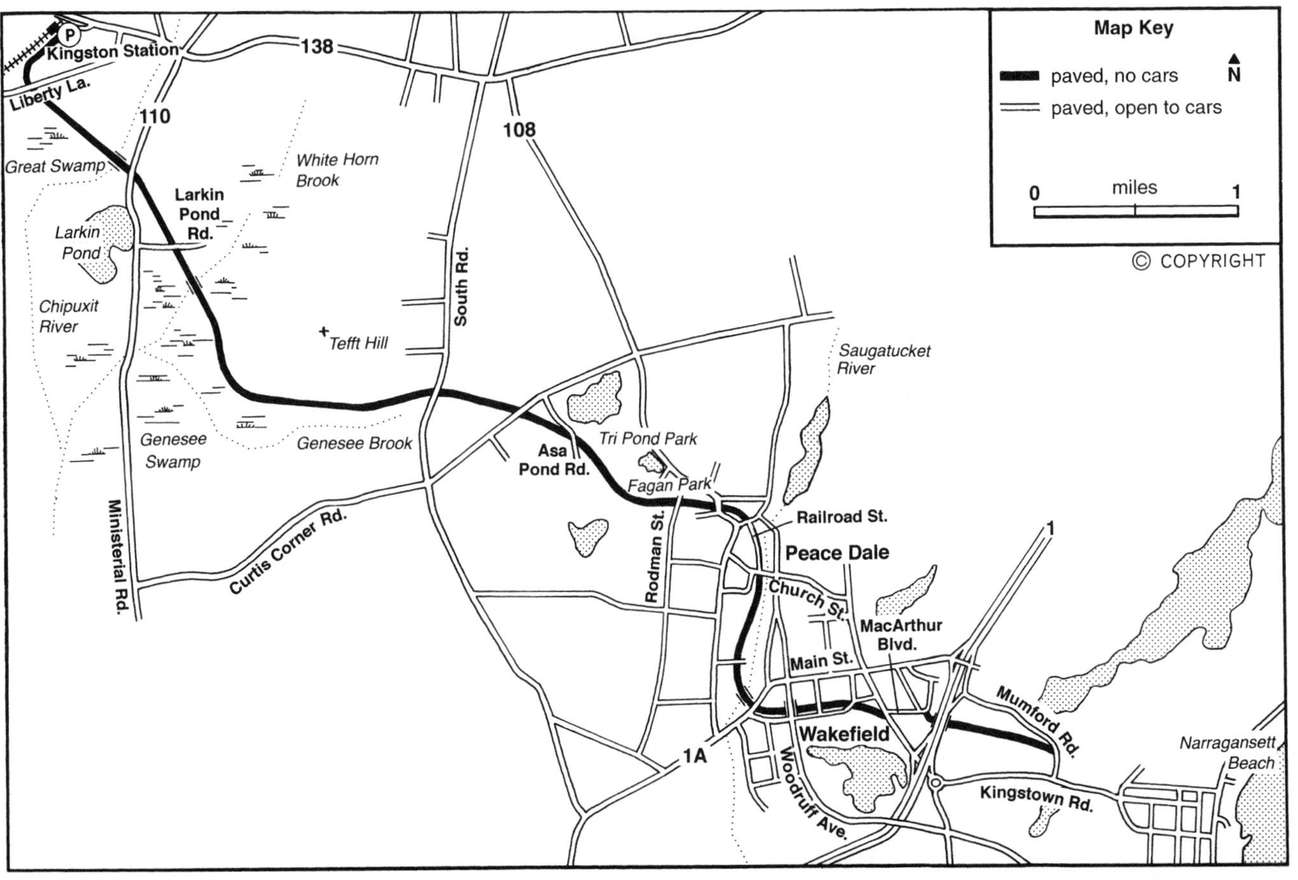

Map Key
paved, no cars
paved, open to cars
N
0
miles
1
© COPYRIGHT
Kingston Station
P
Liberty La.
138
110
108
Great Swamp
White Horn Brook
Larkin Pond Rd.
Larkin Pond
Chipuxit River
South Rd.
Tefft Hill
Genesee Swamp
Genesee Brook
Ministerial Rd.
Curtis Corner Rd.
Asa Pond Rd.
Tri Pond Park
Fagan Park
Saugatucket River
Railroad St.
Rodman St.
Peace Dale
Church St.
MacArthur Blvd.
Main St.
1
Wakefield
1A
Woodruff Ave.
Mumford Rd.
Kingstown Rd.
Narragansett Beach

road bike route extends from the eastern terminus to Narragansett Beach.

TRAIL DESCRIPTION:

Start at the trail's western end at **Kingston Station** on **Rte. 138**. Beginning from the southwestern end of the parking lot, the bike path curves past industrial buildings near the intersection of **Liberty La.** and then heads southeast into natural surroundings. The 3,300-acre **Great Swamp Wildlife Management Area** preserves the wetland and forest scenery on the right (southwest) side of the trail and farm fields are visible through trees on the left. Ahead, a view awaits at a bridge over the **Chipuxit River**.

The bike path intersects **Ministerial Rd.** (**Rte. 110**) after 0.9 miles and then **Larkin Pond Rd.** before emerging in the open area of **Genesee Swamp** which provides interesting scenery on both sides. Halfway across, it passes over a bridge on **White Horn Brook**.

Returning to woods on the other side, the bike path turns eastward as it rounds the base of **Tefft Hill** and follows the valley of **Genesee Brook** where wild rhododendrons and mountain laurels grow in the shade of the forest. It intersects **South Rd.** (2.9 miles), **Curtis Corner Rd.** (3.3 miles) beside a school, and **Asa Pond Rd.** (3.6 miles) before returning to natural environs. **Tri Pond Park**, a town-owned preserve, surrounds the next leg with more wetland scenery.

The trail reaches **Fagan Park** at 4.2 miles where a small playground, a water fountain, and picnic table invite a rest. Just ahead, it intersects **Rodman St.** (4.3 miles) and approaches the village of **Peace Dale** where it descends a slope in sharp switchback turns to the first crossing of busy **Rte. 108** (4.5 miles) where a bridge once carried the railroad over the road. It soon crosses Rte. 108 a second time, then continues straight on **Railroad St.** and begins a 0.2-mile on-road leg which has little car traffic. Turning south, the road passes the village's former train station and then ends at **Church St.** where the separated bike path resumes.

The bike path follows the edge of Riverside

Cemetery for much of the next half-mile, crosses a bridge over the **Saugatucket River** (5.5 miles), and curves back to the east as it intersects **Main St.** (**Rte 1A**) (5.6 miles) in the busy commercial area of **Wakefield**. A cluster of roads in the next half-mile brings the trail under **Woodruff Ave.**, across Prospect Ave., and across Robinson St. before it passes behind a shopping center to reach the third and final crossing of Rte. 108 (6.3 miles).

A signal and crosswalk guide trail travelers across the busy road and signs mark a second on-road leg continuing straight ahead on **MacArthur Blvd.**, another quiet residential street. After 0.2 miles, look for the separated bike path on the right just before the road curves to the left.

The trail curves downhill to join the original railroad grade and enters a tunnel beneath **Rte. 1** where a designated "tunnel gallery" exhibits municipally approved graffiti art. Straightening, the trail levels in a wooded area, hits the Narragansett town line, and ends at **Mumford Rd.**, 7.2 miles from Kingston Station.

For an ocean view, bicyclists can continue along a marked route on roads for 1.2 miles to **Narragansett Beach**. Following green *Bike Route* signs, turn right on Mumford Rd. at the end of the bike path and ride for 0.3 miles, then turn left on **Kingstown Rd.** Keep straight at the next four-way intersection where Kingstown Rd. turns right and follow Narragansett Ave. straight to the end at a T-intersection. Turn left on Narragansett Ave. and follow it for a quarter-mile to the end.

BACKGROUND:

This route originated in 1876 as the Narragansett Railroad. Built primarily to provide freight service between the textile mills at Peace Dale and Wakefield and the nearby port of Narragansett Pier, the line also came to serve significant passenger service for the growing summer tourist trade at Narragansett Beach in the 1890's. A slow decline in the 1900's saw passenger service on the line end in 1952 and freight service end in 1968.

After years of dormancy, proposals to create a multi-use trail produced results. The bike path was constructed in phases in 2000, 2003, and 2011, and future construction is being designed. The bike path is named in honor of State Senator William C. O'Neill, one of the trail's earliest advocates.

DRIVING DIRECTIONS:

From I-95 take Exit 3 and follow Rte. 138 east for 8.2 miles. After crossing a bridge over railroad tracks, turn left following signs to Kingston Station. Park at the far (south) end of the lot, where the bike path begins.

From Rte. 1 in South Kingstown, turn west on Rte. 138 and drive for about 6 miles. Follow signs to Kingston Station just before the road rises and passes over the railroad tracks. Park at the far (south) end of the lot, where the bike path begins.

TOILETS:

Kingston Station, Narragansett Town Beach

ADDITIONAL INFORMATION:

South Kingstown Parks & Recreation Dept., (401) 789-9301
Friends of the William C. O'Neill Bike Path,
www.southcountybikepath.org

39 Quonset Bike Path

North Kingstown, RI

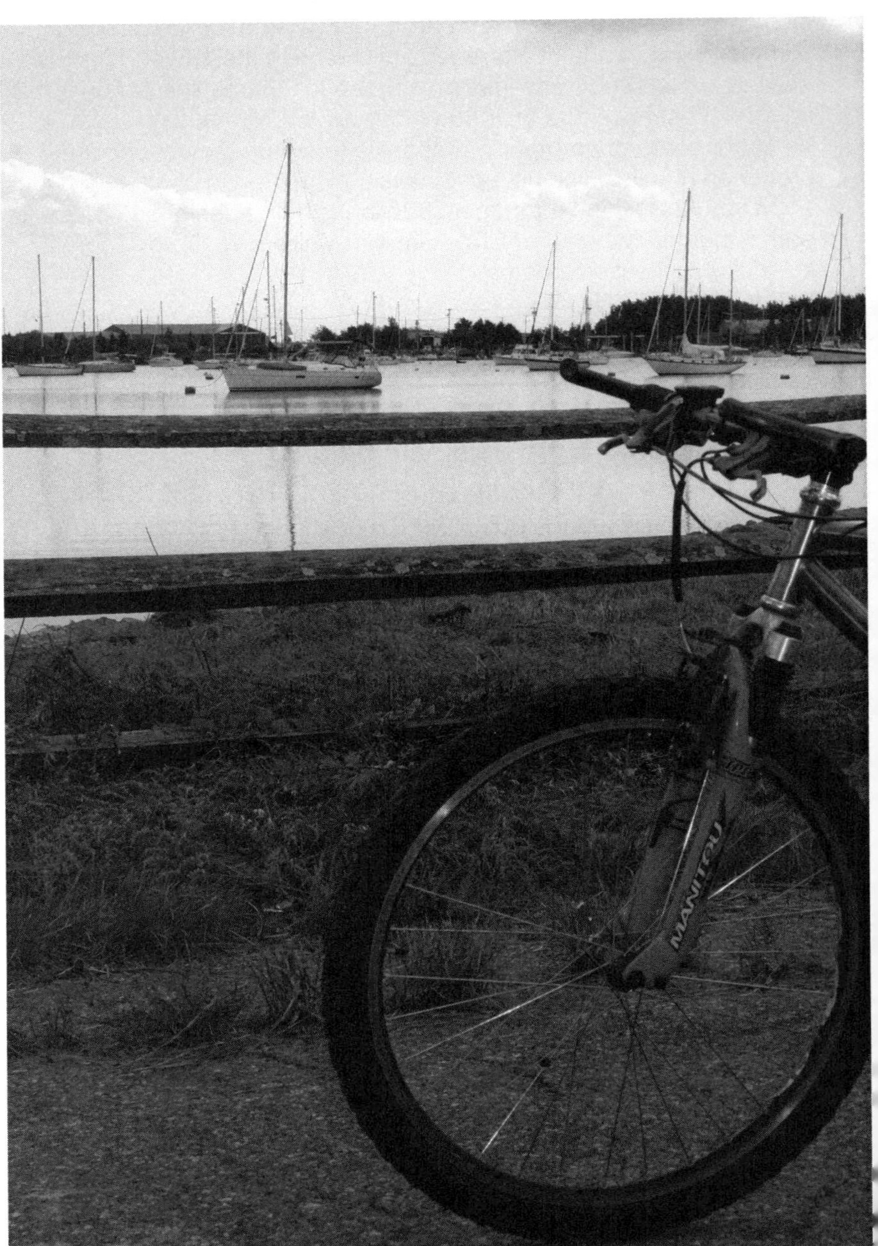

LENGTH: 3.8 miles
SURFACE: paved
TERRAIN: gentle slopes

This former military base, birthplace of the Quonset Hut, has been redeveloped with a bike path running along its perimeter to a Narragansett Bay beach. The biking is free of any road intersections and well suited for a ride with kids.

RULES & SAFETY:

• Bicyclists should yield to pedestrians.

• Keep to the right, pass on the left, and alert others (*"On your left..."*) when approaching from behind.

• Note that walkers are requested to use the left side.

• Ride at a safe speed, and use extra caution when children and pets are present since their movements can be unpredictable.

• Dogs must be leashed and their wastes removed.

• The area is open from dawn to dusk.

ORIENTATION:

The bike path extends from Rte. 1 in the southwest to Narragansett Bay in the northeast, with a trailhead parking lot in the middle. In general, scenery is most interesting along the northeast section of the trail although its paved surface is the remains of an old road and is crumbling and overgrown in places. In contrast, the southwest section has relatively bland scenery but its trail surface is new and generously landscaped with trees, shrubs, and mowed grass. The trail has several points of access from nearby roads.

TRAIL DESCRIPTION:

Heading southwest from the **Marine Rd.** trailhead, the bike path runs for 2.5 miles along the perimeter of the former military base. Ride back to the curve in the road (heading west) and fork right on the bike path. It begins with a 0.6-mile straight line course through woods to an intersection of nearby residential streets where a paved side trail connects the neighborhood. It then curves left (south) and continues beside woods paralleling **Newcomb Rd.** for a half-mile.

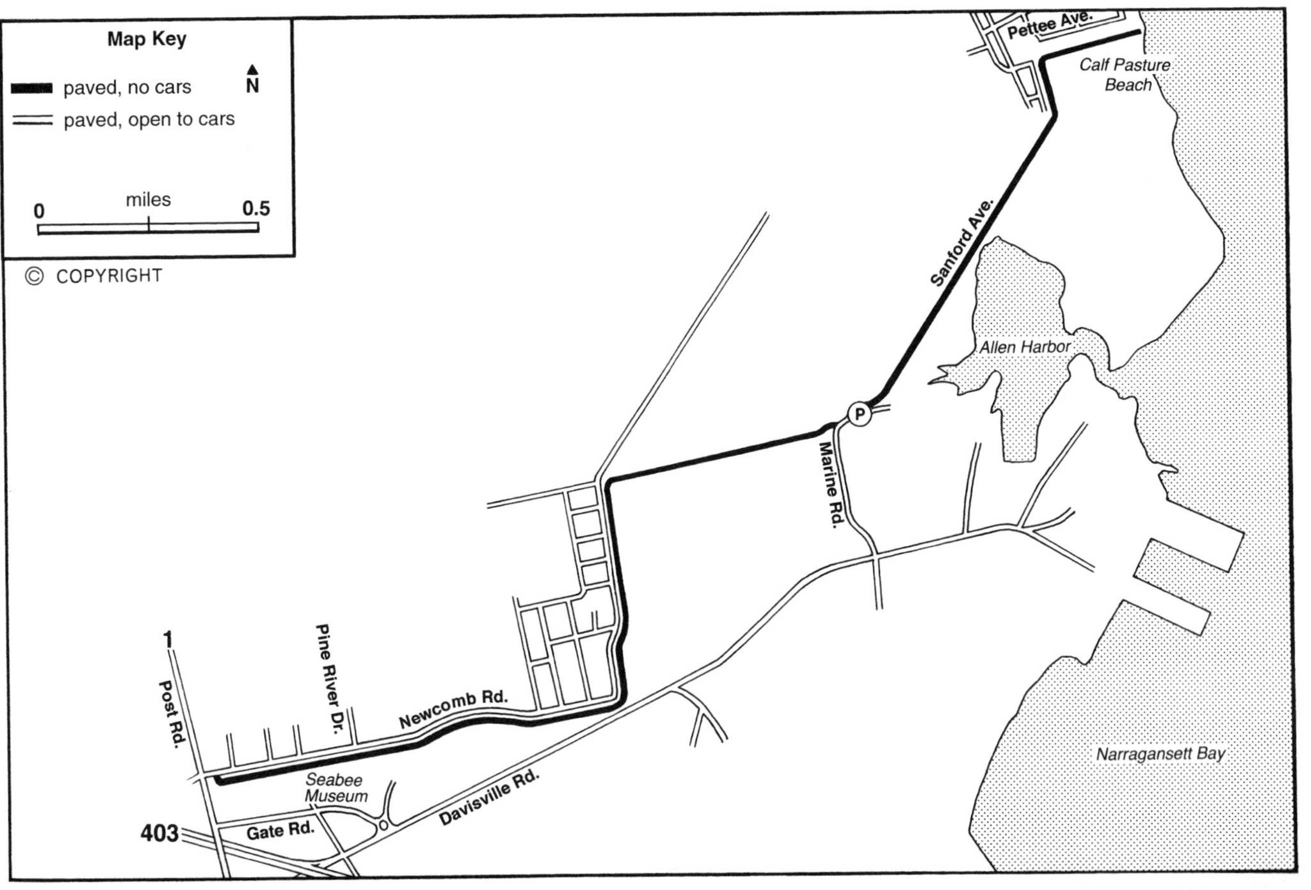
Map Key
paved, no cars
paved, open to cars
N
0
miles
0.5
© COPYRIGHT
Pettee Ave.
Calf Pasture Beach
Sanford Ave.
Allen Harbor
P
Marine Rd.
Narragansett Bay
1
Post Rd.
Pine River Dr.
Newcomb Rd.
Seabee Museum
Gate Rd.
403
Davisville Rd.

Just before reaching **Davisville Rd.**, it leaves the cover of trees and curves back to the right (west) alongside Newcomb Rd. in open surroundings. An earthen banking shields the bike path from a shopping center on the left while fencing separates the nearby roadway on the right.

After a connection to **Pine River Dr.** on the right, the trail comes beside woods and passes the **Seabee Museum and Memorial Park** just before a department store on the left side, then ends a quarter-mile ahead at Newcomb Rd. near its intersection with **Rte. 1** (**Post Rd.**).

Heading northeast from the trailhead on Marine Rd., bicyclists can ride for 1.3 miles on the remains of **Sanford Ave.** and enjoy more natural scenery. Although it's cracking with age and overgrowing in places, the road allows smooth rolling as it continues straight off the end of the parking lot past a metal gate blocking vehicles. It passes the edge of **Allen Harbor** on the right after a half-mile and later parallels **Pettee Ave.** before ending at **Calf Pasture Beach** and a view of **Narragansett Bay**.

BACKGROUND:

In the early 1940's, the U.S. Military developed this land into the Davisville Seabee Complex utilizing about 3,000 acres for various purposes. One such use was a training center for the Navy's Seabees, a construction force which built facilities to support the war effort. One of the base's most lasting creations was the Quonset Hut, an arched-roof structure which could be quickly and easily shipped to distant lands and be erected to house personnel and materials. The Quonset Hut took its name from a Native American word given to a nearby point of land in Narragansett Bay. The Seabee Museum on Gate Rd. preserves the former base's history.

The property is being redeveloped as the Quonset Business Park with some areas preserved as open space. The bike path was completed in 2009.

DRIVING DIRECTIONS:

From Rte. 4 take Exit 7 and follow Rte. 403 south for 2.3 miles to the Davisville Rd. exit. Follow Davisville Rd. for 1.5 miles, turn left on Marine Rd., and park at the end.

TOILETS:

none on site

40 Warwick City Park Bike Path

Warwick, RI

LENGTH: 2.8 miles
SURFACE: paved
TERRAIN: small hills

Warwick City Park is a 200-acre recreation area on a peninsula in Greenwich Bay complete with a beach, a playground, and an array of athletic fields. Its lively bike path offers pretty water views as it rolls and curves through woods along the shoreline.

RULES & SAFETY:

- The bike path loop is to be ridden one-way in the clockwise direction.
- Bicyclists are requested to keep to the right side, and walkers and runners are to use the left side.
- The bike path is hilly and curvy so ride at a safe speed.
- Use extra caution when children and pets are present since their movements can be unpredictable.
- Remember that fallen leaves are slippery when wet.
- Watch for thorn bushes overhanging the trail.
- Alert others when approaching from behind to avoid startling them.
- Dogs must be leashed and their wastes removed.
- Parking is allowed only in designated areas. Avoid leaving valuables locked in your car.
- The park is open from sunrise to sunset.

ORIENTATION:

The bike path forms a one-way loop (to be ridden in the clockwise direction) along the park's periphery, following the shoreline for most of the way. Road intersections occur at three locations but car traffic is minimal.

The paved surface is in good condition and has a painted dividing line to separate bicyclists from walkers.

Mileage markers are posted at half-mile intervals and benches are provided at numerous places. Several parking lots provide options for starting points along the loop, but visitors should note that the beach and the playing field lots can sometimes be crowded.

TRAIL DESCRIPTION:

Begin at the **main gate** where a trailhead parking lot and maintenance building mark the start of the loop. Follow the paved pathway beside **Steven O'Connor Blvd.**, the park's entrance roadway, past the gate at the stone wall, then fork left in the clockwise direction.

The bike path begins along the edge of a mowed field, turns left into nearby woods, and descends with a switchback to the edge of **Brush Neck Cove**. Heading east along the water, the paved trail curves through oak forest on a hilly course for over a mile with a few bigger slopes near the midpoint. Trees block some of the views but openings between branches allow glimpses over the water to residential neighborhoods on the opposite shore. Watch for overhanging thorn bushes along this stretch since they can threaten both skin and bicycle tires.

Before the half-mile mark the bike path intersects a paved side trail on the right which makes a short-cut in the loop and connects Steven O'Connor Blvd. at a small trail-head parking area.

The terrain gets milder and the viewpoints become more frequent as the bike path approaches the end of the peninsula. Turning southwest, the trail intersects the park's roadway near the 1.3-mile mark where a large parking lot serves **Raymond Stone Beach**, the park's highlight during the warm summer months. For a short side-trip, turn left into the parking lot and continue to the water's edge where the view extends southward across Greenwich Bay to Narragansett Bay. Toilets are open at this location during the swimming season.

Continuing on the loop, the bike path intersects the park's roadway a second time at the 1.4-mile mark. It turns

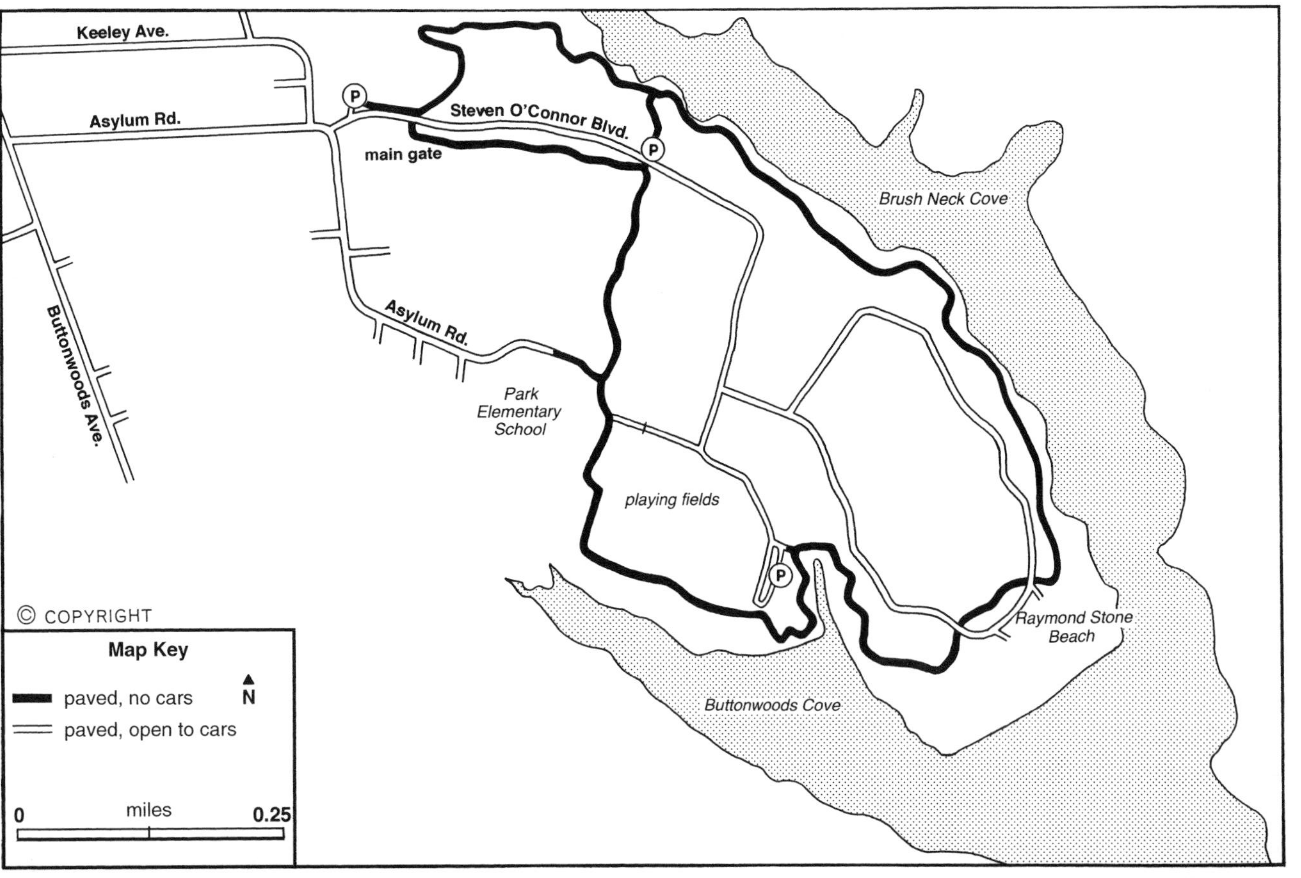

Keeley Ave.
Asylum Rd.
Steven O'Connor Blvd.
main gate
Brush Neck Cove
Buttonwoods Ave.
Asylum Rd.
Park Elementary School
playing fields
Raymond Stone Beach
Buttonwoods Cove
P
P
P
© COPYRIGHT
Map Key
paved, no cars
paved, open to cars
N
0
miles
0.25

westward at the edge of **Buttonwoods Cove** and, after curving around a small inlet in the shoreline, emerges at an open area of **playing fields** and another trailhead parking lot. It follows the perimeter of the fields for the next half-mile, turning north and passing a side trail to **Park Elementary School** along the way.

Returning to shade at the 2.3-mile mark, the bike path curves through a stand of pitch pines for a short distance before returning to the edge of Steven O'Connor Blvd., where it intersects the short-cut trail. The last quarter-mile heads west paralleling the roadway back to the entrance gate.

BACKGROUND:

Also known as Brush Neck, this peninsula came to be the site of the Warwick Asylum, or poor farm, which was built in 1870 to house the city's citizens who were in need of assistance. Residents used the property to grow crops and raise livestock until 1940 when the asylum was closed. The buildings were dismantled in the 1950's and the property has been gradually developed for recreational purposes since that time.

DRIVING DIRECTIONS:

From I-95 southbound take Exit 10A and follow Rte. 117 east for 2.5 miles, or from **I-95 northbound** take Exit 10 and follow Rte. 117 east for 2.1 miles. At a traffic signal and shopping center, turn right on Buttonwoods Ave. and drive for 0.4 miles, turn left on Aylum Rd. and continue for 0.3 miles, then turn left at the park entrance. Either park at the trailhead on the left at the main gate or locate other parking lots on the trail map.

TOILETS:

Raymond Stone Beach during the swimming season.

ADDITIONAL INFORMATION:

Warwick City Park, (401) 738-2000

41 Fred Lippitt Woonasquatucket River Greenway

Providence - Johnston, RI

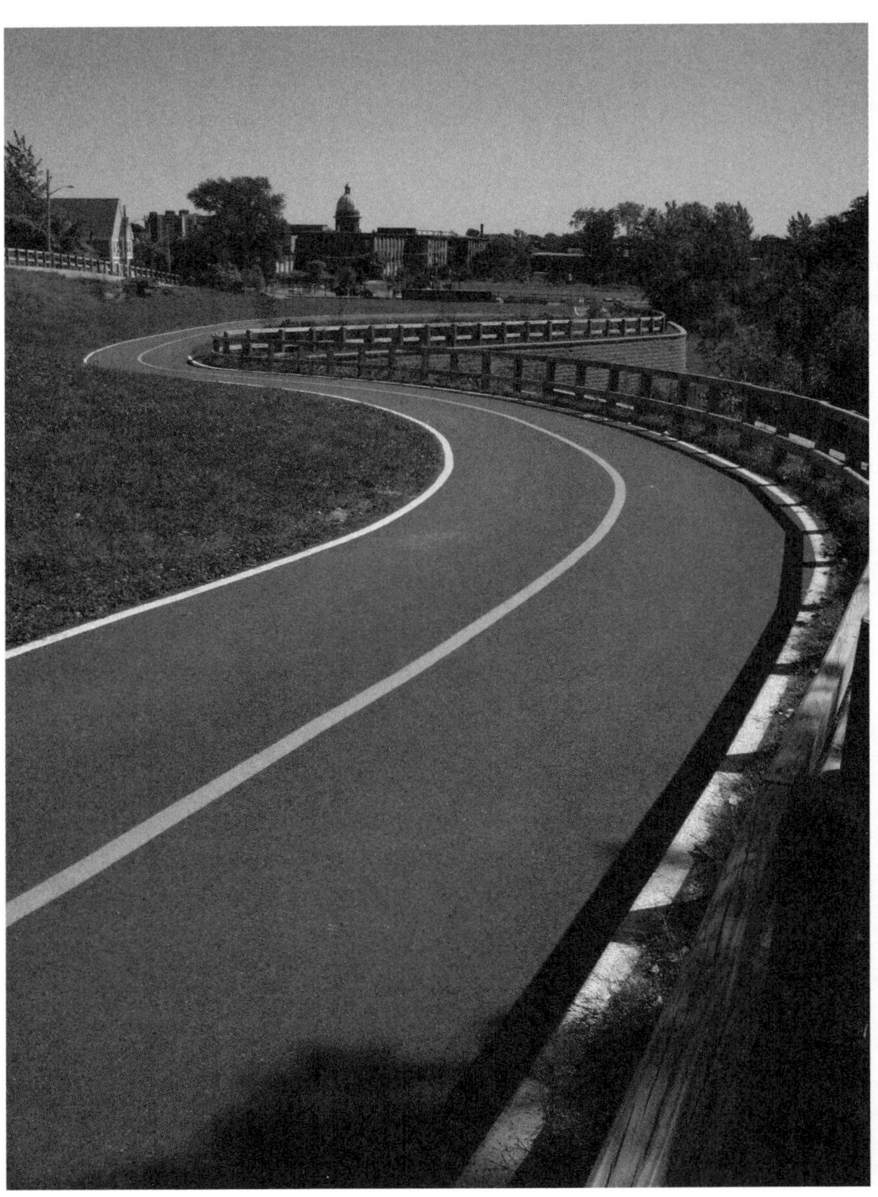

LENGTH: 2.4 miles, plus side trails
SURFACE: paved
TERRAIN: mostly flat, some slopes at the south end

A true greenway, this short rail-trail has brought welcome progress to the Woonasquatucket River and the surrounding community, and enables bicyclists and walkers to enjoy the natural scenery while avoiding the area's cramped streets.

RULES & SAFETY:

- Bicyclists should yield to pedestrians.
- Keep to the right, pass on the left, and alert others (*"On your left..."*) when approaching from behind.
- Ride at a safe speed and be especially cautious in the presence of children and pets since their movements can be unpredictable.
- Help keep the area clean by carrying out at least as much as you carry in.
- Dogs must be leashed and their wastes removed.

ORIENTATION:

The Fred Lippitt Woonasquatucket River Greenway extends along the Woonasquatucket River from Providence in the southeast to Johnston in the northwest. Side trails intersect at a few points along the greenway to connect surrounding neighborhoods.

Trailhead parking is provided at two locations shown on the map, with the largest being Marino Park which is located at the south end of the greenway and linked by a side trail.

TRAIL DESCRIPTION:

Begin in Providence at **Merino Park** where a pedestrian bridge rises on a ramp from the parking area to span both **Rte. 6** and the **Woonasquatucket River** and reach the rail-trail on the other side. Turning to the right (southeast), the greenway trail descends in curves for a short distance to **Riverside Mills Park** off **Aleppo St.** in **Olneyville**, where the pathway ends at an open area of

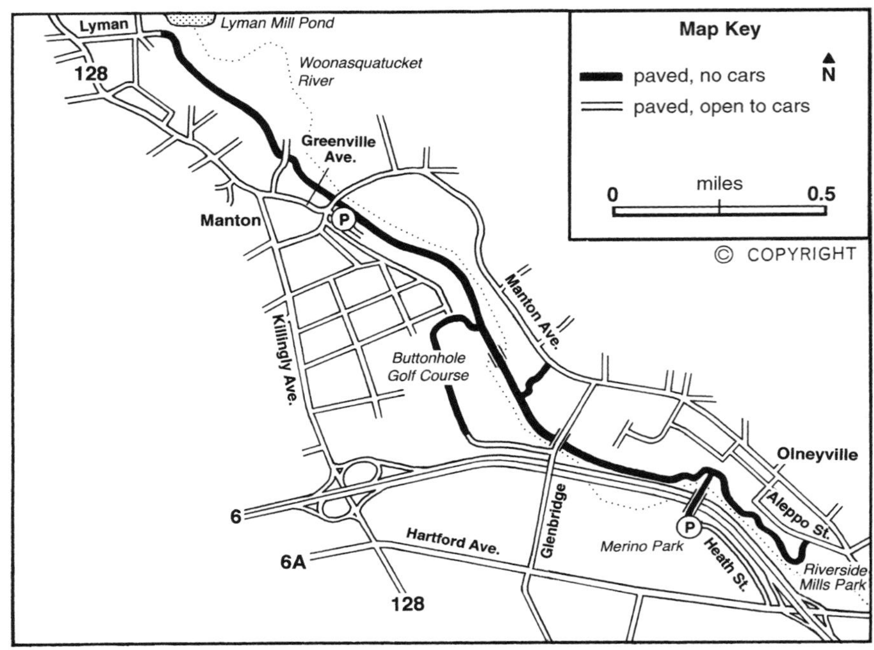

lawn, a playground, and stone benches beside the river. A marked, on-road bike route continues from this point into the city.

Turning to the left (northwest) from the Merino Park pedestrian bridge, the trail currently extends for 2 miles with enjoyable scenery along the Woonasquatucket. It joins the side of Rte 6 for a quarter-mile before veering northward on a separate, quieter course along the river, passing under a bridge carrying **Glenbridge Ave.** along the way. Just ahead, it intersects a side trail on the right which climbs a strenuous slope for three quarters of a mile to **Manton Ave.**

Continuing on the greenway, quiet, shady conditions bring the trail past the **Buttonhole Golf Course** on the left. After the trail crosses a bridge over the river and enters Johnston, it intersects another side trail on the left which circles the northern fringe of the golf course and links its entrance driveway.

A half-mile north, the trail comes beside a small trailhead parking area and intersects **Greenville Ave.** at the village of **Manton**, 1.3 miles from the Merino Park bridge.

Fencing, plantings, and mowed grass border the trail as it passes a mix of industrial, residential, and natural areas along the last 0.7-mile leg. It starts beside the river for a quarter-mile, then crosses a private road and continues for another half-mile to the current northern terminus at the end of **Lyman Ave.** where a view of **Lyman Mill Pond** extends to the north. No parking is available at this endpoint.

BACKGROUND:

The trail follows the route of the Providence & Springfield Railroad which was completed between Olneyville and Pascoag in 1873 and extended into Providence in 1874. It remained only a branch line until 1893 when the New York and New England Railroad extended it to reach another rail line at Douglas, MA. The railroad achieved modest success with passenger service to and from the city and with freight service from a few textile mills along the route but was never able to serve its intended destination of Springfield, MA. Passenger service on the line ended during the Great Depression and freight service continued until the 1960's.

Its redevelopment as a recreational greenway was initiated in 1993 by Fred Lippitt, chairman of the Providence Plan, as part of a greater effort to restore the river and improve surrounding neighborhoods. The work has included restoring wetlands, cleaning up former industrial sites, and developing affordable housing. The bike path was dedicated in 2007, and additional construction is expected to extend it northward in future years.

DRIVING DIRECTIONS:

From I-95 take Exit 22B and follow Rte. 6 west for 1.8 miles. After the split with Rte. 10, take the Rte. 6A/Hartford Ave. exit and turn left off the ramp heading west. Proceed under the highway then turn immediately right on Heath St. and continue to the end at Marino Park. Take the pedestrian bridge over Rte. 6 to reach the greenway.

TOILETS:

none are provided

ADDITIONAL INFORMATION:

Woonasquatucket River Watershed Council, wrwc.org/greenway

42 Blackstone River Bikeway

Cumberland - Woonsocket, RI

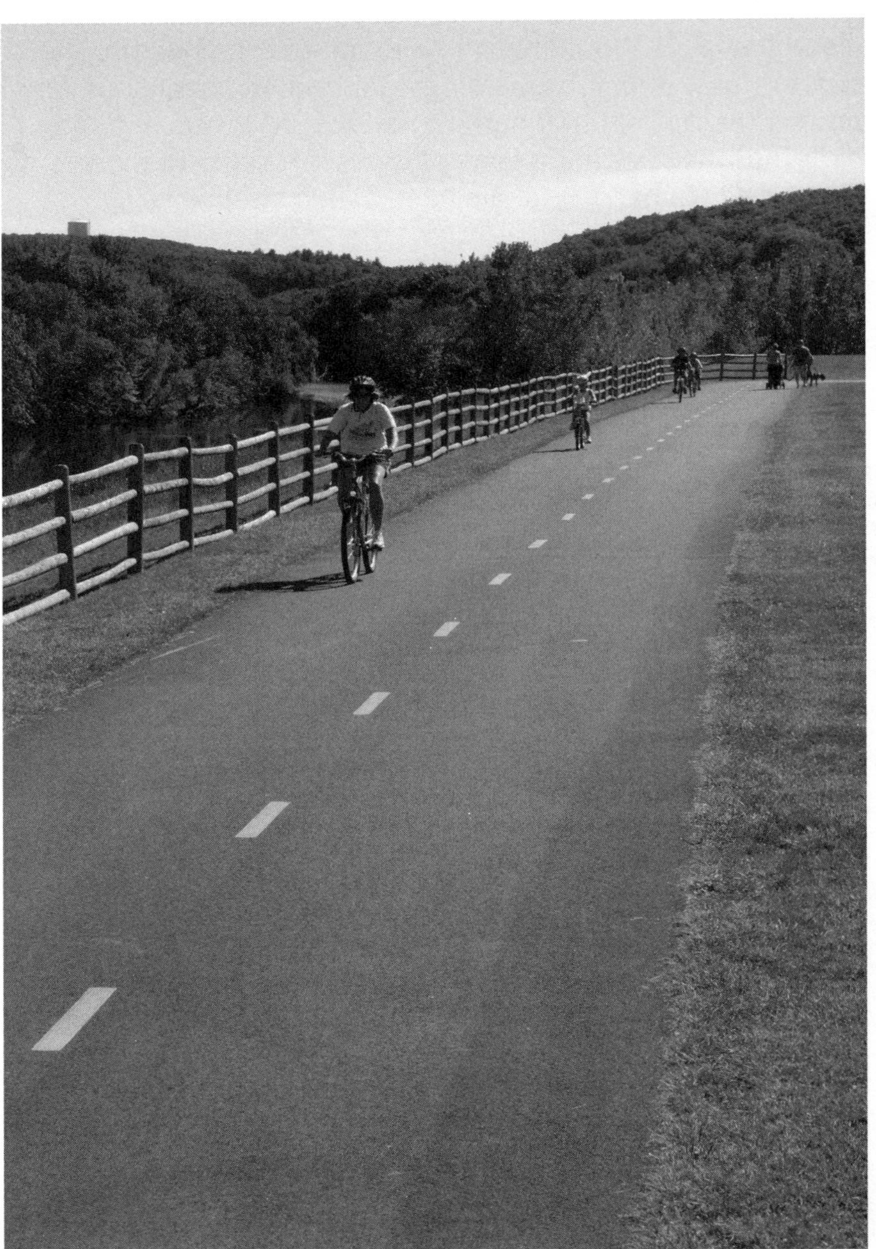

LENGTH: 10 miles, plus side trails
SURFACE: paved
TERRAIN: gentle slopes

Following the Blackstone River, this famous bike path threads an impressive route along a historic canal, past old mill villages, and through protected natural areas. Amazingly, the trail crosses traffic at only 3 intersections.

RULES & SAFETY:

- Bicyclists should yield to pedestrians.
- Keep to the right, pass on the left, and alert others when approaching from behind to avoid startling them.
- Note that walkers are requested to use the left side.
- Step off the trail when stopped to allow others to pass.
- Ride at a safe speed, and use extra caution in crowded areas and when children and pets are present since their movements can be unpredictable.
- Respect the private property along the trail.
- Help keep it clean by carrying out all that you carry in.
- Dogs must be leashed and their wastes removed.
- The trail is open from sunrise to sunset.

ORIENTATION:

Confined by a river, canal, railroad, and nearby streets, the Blackstone River Bikeway contends with a variety of conditions involving small hills, sharp turns, numerous bridges, and even its own railroad crossing.

Several spur trails branch from the bikeway to reach nearby trailhead parking lots. It should be noted that the two that intersect under the Rte. 116 bridge climb significant hills (in switchbacks, so the slope is manageable) before reaching the parking lots at the I-295 visitor center and at Rte. 116. Other trailheads exist near each of the bikeway's endpoints and at points in between.

Natural scenery lies along the entire length of the trail, but the northernmost 6 miles follow railroad tracks closely; fortunately, trains are infrequent. Granite mileage markers placed at half-mile intervals along the trail originate in

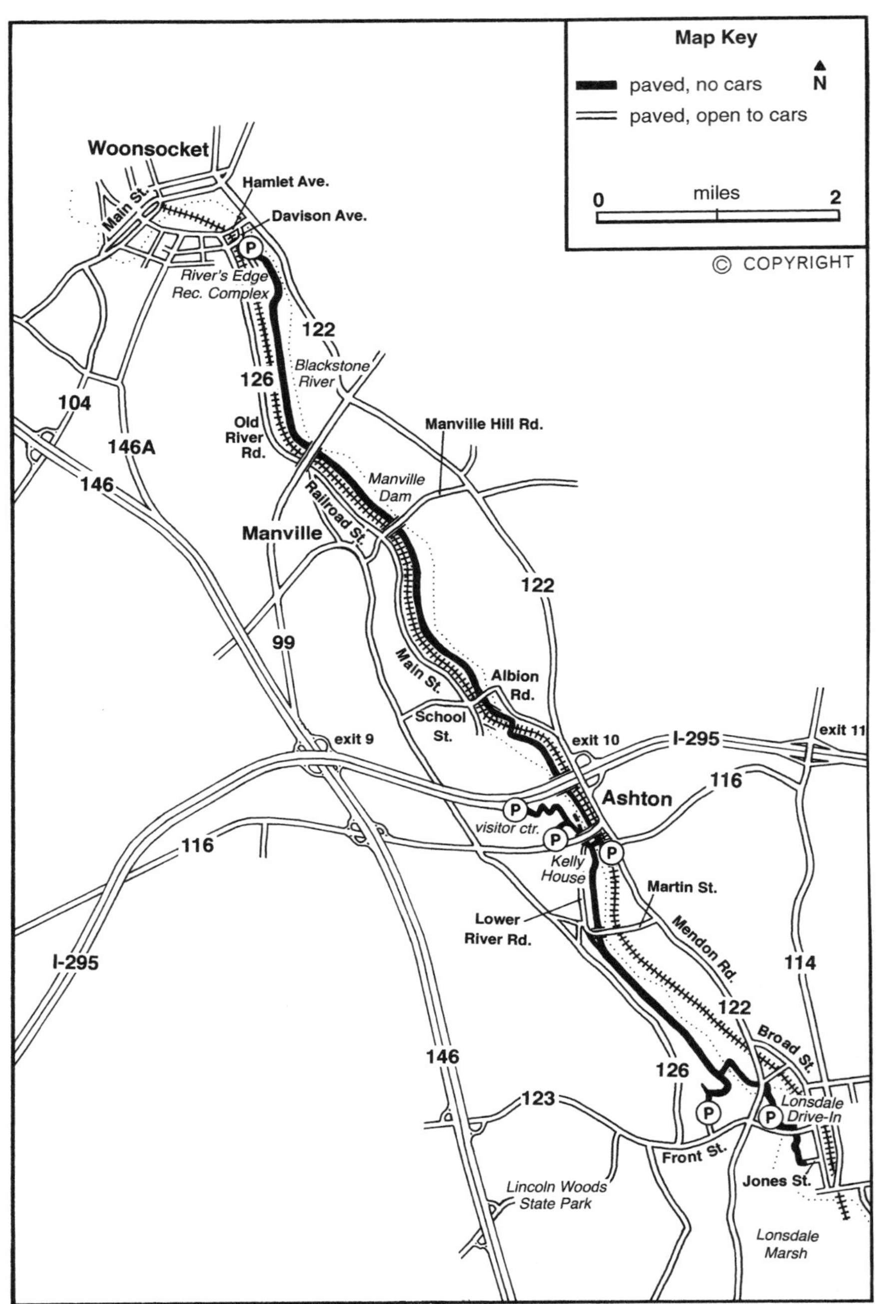
Map Key
paved, no cars
paved, open to cars
N
0
miles
2
© COPYRIGHT
Woonsocket
Main St.
Hamlet Ave.
Davison Ave.
River's Edge
Rec. Complex
122
Blackstone
River
126
104
146A
Old
River
Rd.
Manville Hill Rd.
146
Manville
Dam
Manville
Railroad St.
122
99
Main St.
Albion
Rd.
School
St.
exit 9
exit 10
I-295
exit 11
Ashton
116
visitor ctr.
116
Kelly
House
Martin St.
Lower
River Rd.
Mendon Rd.
I-295
114
122
Broad St.
146
126
123
Lonsdale
Drive-In
Front St.
Jones St.
Lincoln Woods
State Park
Lonsdale
Marsh

Providence. Green *Bike Route* signs guide trail travelers through intersections and other potential points of confusion, and historical information is displayed at several places along the way.

TRAIL DESCRIPTION:

Starting in Lincoln at the **Lonsdale Drive-In** trailhead near the southern end of the bikeway, the trail extends in two directions. Heading south it runs for a half-mile, crossing **Rte. 123** and entering **Lonsdale Marsh** in Cumberland with a long boardwalk before ending at **Jones St.** A marked, on-road bike route continues southward from this point into Providence.

Heading north, the trail continues for 9.5 miles. It skirts the clearing of the former Lonsdale Drive-In Theatre, shares a bridge over the **Blackstone River** with **Rte. 122**, then crosses the busy road at a traffic signal (0.4 miles). The trail continues through trees along wooden fencing, turns sharply left and crosses back over the river on a former railroad bridge, and forks on the other side (0.9 miles). A short spur on the left connects a trailhead parking lot off **Front St.** while the main trail turns right (north).

Here it begins a 2-mile leg along the original towpath for the Blackstone Canal, which provides an enjoyable water view along the way. The river parallels on the other side of the trail and is visible at several points.

The trail passes under the **Martin St.** bridge (2.5 miles), then turns off the towpath at the 2.9-mile mark and circles a meadow before reaching a trail intersection beneath the **Rte. 116** bridge (3.4 miles) at the **Kelly House** Museum which houses historical displays for the canal and surrounding mills.

Here a few side trails fork left as the main bikeway turns hard right to cross the river. Straight ahead, an unpaved spur continues upstream for a quarter-mile. To the left, a paved trail crosses the canal and climbs a hill to reach two trailhead parking lots: fork left to reach the Rte. 116 trail-head or fork right to climb a bigger hill to the **I-295 Visitor**

Center (0.9 miles from the canal) where toilets are located.

Continuing northward on the bikeway, the trail enters Cumberland as it crosses a large bridge over the Blackstone River to the brick mill buildings of **Ashton** and turns left (north) alongside the Providence & Worcester Railroad which it follows for the next 6 miles. It passes under twin bridges for **I-295** a half-mile ahead, then intersects the railroad (4.6 miles) at a unique "bikeway crossing" point complete with its own gates and signals. The trail crosses the river again, returns to the town of Lincoln, and intersects **Albion Rd.** near the 5-mile mark at another old brick mill building.

Upstream, the bikeway follows the river closely with water views on the right side relieving the sight of the railroad and its chainlink fencej on the left. The bikeway passes a small trailhead parking lot off **New River Rd.** before reaching the village of **Manville** where it passes under a bridge for **Manville Hill Rd.** and gets a view of the **Manville Dam** (6.7 miles), the Blackstone's biggest with an 18' drop.

The trail progresses along a narrow corridor between the river and the railroad with sections of the old canal bed appearing as well. A mile ahead, the river valley constricts and turns amid surrounding hills as the bikeway passes under a high bridge carrying **Rte. 99**. It hits the Woonsocket city line (7.8 miles) just beyond this point, gets a narrower trail surface as it passes a water treatment facility, then rises on an uphill slope to the **Rivers Edge Recreation Complex** (9.1 miles) where playing fields provide a vast open area. Once a landfill, this high ground overlooks the river and, together with its trailhead parking, toilet facilities, and snack bar, now makes a popular attraction along the bikeway.

Following wooden fencing around the edge of the recreation area, the trail descends to the park's entrance drive and follows it to another trailhead parking lot at **Davison Ave.** where the separated pathway currently ends, 9.5 miles north of the Lonsdale Drive-In trailhead.

BACKGROUND:

The bikeway follows the Blackstone Canal which was dug by shovel and cart between Providence and Worcester, MA in 1828. A stimulus for commerce, the canal provided efficient transportaton for farmers and manufacturers to ship goods until the arrival of the Providence & Worcester Railroad in 1847 when it became obsolete.

During the Industrial Revolution, dams built along the Blackstone River harnessed its energy to power textile mills which employed thousands of workers in the production of cotton and woolen materials. By 1880, the Blackstone was hailed *the hardest working river* as a result of the intense industrial exploitation along its course.

The John H. Chafee Blackstone River Valley National Heritage Corridor was created by Congress in 1986 to preserve this history. Extending 45 miles from Providence to Worcester, the corridor's centerpiece will be the Blackstone River Bikeway, a mostly off-road accessible trail designed to link the area's significant natural and historic features with an enjoyable place to walk and ride. Trail construction has progressed in phases, with 10 miles completed in Rhode Island and a 2.3-mile segment open in Massachusetts. The bikeway serves as an important part of the East Coast Greenway, a trail being created between Maine and Florida.

DRIVING DIRECTIONS:

Lonsdale Drive-In, Lincoln: From I-295, take Exit 10 and follow Rte. 122 south for 3.3 miles. Turn left on Rte. 123 and look for the trailhead entrance at the *Lonsdale Drive-In* sign a short distance ahead on the left.

Rte. 116, Lincoln: From I-295, take Exit 10 and follow Rte. 122 south for 0.5 miles. Turn right on Rte. 116 west and continue for 0.2 miles to the trailhead on the right.

I-295 Visitor Center, Lincoln: Northbound between exits 9 and 10. A paved trail connects it to the bikeway, but it requires a considerable uphill return ride.

Davison Ave., Woonsocket: From I-295, take Exit 10 and follow Rte. 122 north for 5.4 miles. After crossing the Blackstone River on Hamlet Ave., turn left on Davison Ave. and find the trailhead on the left before a railroad bridge.

TOILETS:

I-295 Visitor Center in Lincoln,
Rivers Edge Rec. Complex in Woonsocket

ADDITIONAL INFORMATION:

www.blackstoneriverbikeway.com

43 Ten Mile River Greenway

Pawtucket - East Providence, RI

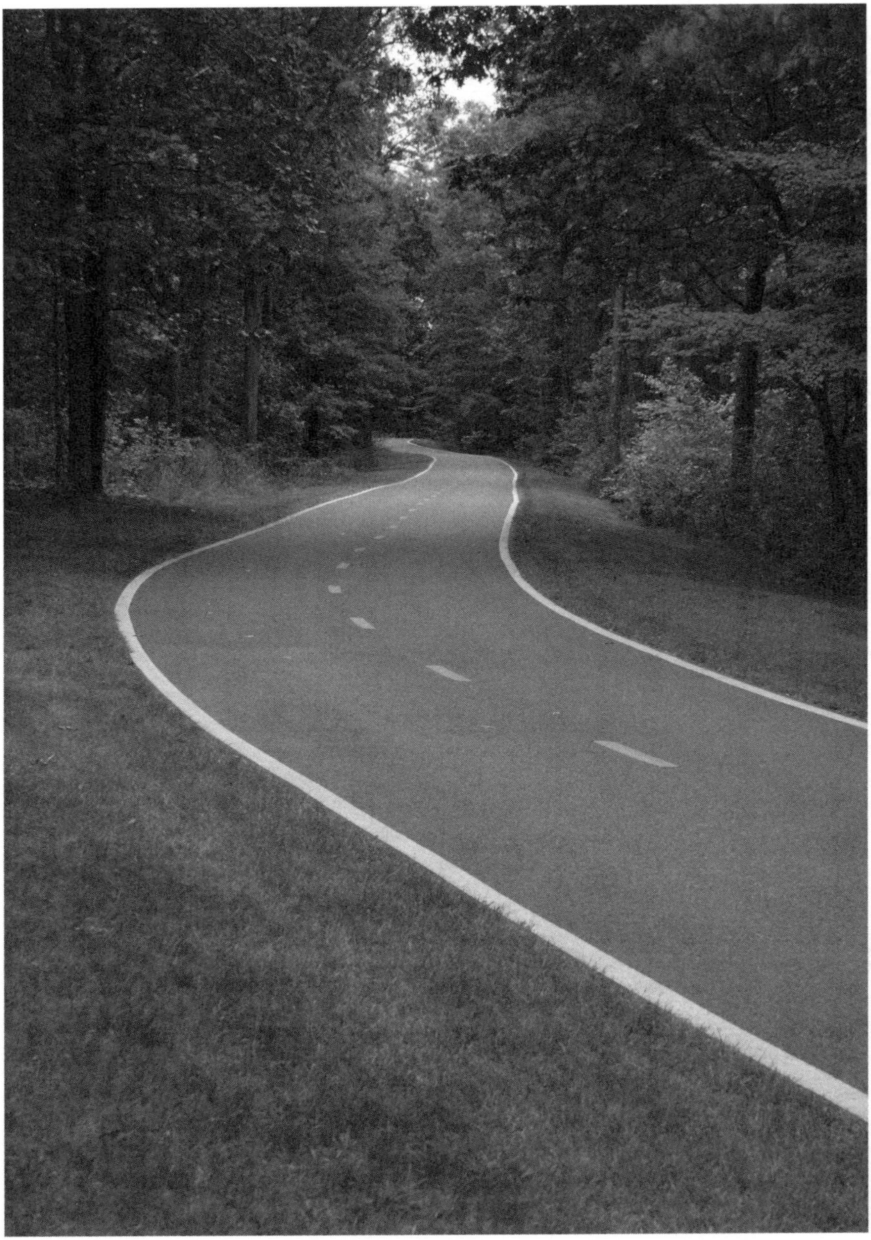

LENGTH: 2.2 miles
SURFACE: paved
TERRAIN: gentle slopes

Not a rail-trail, this rolling, turning, family-friendly pathway joins two parklands with a scenic woodland ride. It has no road intersections so it's a good choice for biking with young children.

RULES & SAFETY:

- Bicyclists should yield to pedestrians.
- Keep to the right, pass on the left, and alert others (*"On your left..."*) when approaching from behind.
- Note that walkers are requested to use the left side.
- Ride at a safe speed and be especially cautious when children and pets are present since their movements can be unpredictable.
- Swimming in the river or the reservoir is not permitted.
- Help keep it clean by carrying out at least as much as you carry in.
- Dogs must be leashed and their wastes removed.
- The trail is open from sunrise to sunset.

ORIENTATION:

Ten Mile River Greenway takes a north-south route from Slater Memorial Park in Pawtucket to Kimberly Ann Rock Memorial Athletic Complex in East Providence. It follows the Ten Mile River for much of the way and, because it intersects no roads, has no other points of access or exit.

Slater Memorial Park is the best starting point and offers picnic areas and toilet facilities in its expansive landscaped grounds which can be explored on bike or foot. The Kimberly Ann Rock Memorial Athletic Complex is another trailhead but can sometimes be busy with sports games.

TRAIL DESCRIPTION:

Begin at the southeast corner of **Slater Memorial Park** where a sharp bend in the perimeter road comes close to the bike path and forms a popular trailhead parking area. To the left, the greenway heads upstream beside **Ten Mile**

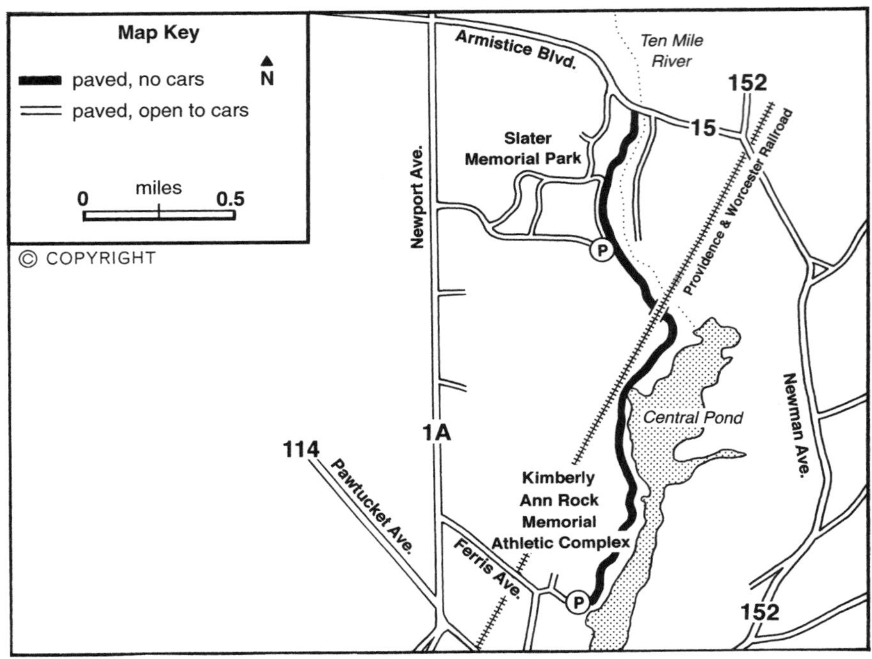

River for 0.6 miles to **Armistice Blvd.**, first in an area of lawns and then curving through woods.

To the right (south), the greenway runs for 1.6 miles. Heading downstream, the trail continues in natural scenery along the river for the first 0.6 miles, passing under the **Providence & Worcester Railroad** along the way. It parallels the railroad tracks at a distance near the north end of **Central Pond**, crosses the East Providence city line, and offers views through trees spreading east over the water. After returning to the edge of the railroad for a short distance, the trail rises on a slope and follows high ground along the western shore for another half-mile with more views of the reservoir filtering through the trees on the left.

The remaining half-mile descends to cross an inlet brook, curves through more woods, and emerges beside the playing fields of the **Kimberly Ann Rock Memorial Athletic Complex** on **Ferris Ave.**, the trail's southern endpoint.

BACKGROUND:

Slater Memorial Park was established in 1894 by the city of Pawtucket and was developed with roads, paths, and athletic fields in the early 1900's. The 200-acre landscaped grounds include a picnic area, playground, and historic 1890's carousel (open during the summer months) and provide a popular complement to the greenway.

The bike path was completed in 2004. Its route utilizes several public lands including Slater Memorial Park in Pawtucket and Kimberly Ann Rock Memorial Athletic Complex in East Providence, as well as acres of former water supply property along Central Pond owned by the city of East Providence. Part of the Turner Reservoir watershed, Central Pond was created in 1930 and used for water supply until 1969.

Future trail construction is planned to extend the greenway north across Armistice Blvd. through the Ten Mile River Reservation to the Daggett Ave. ballfield.

DRIVING DIRECTIONS:

Slater Memorial Park from I-95: Take Exit 2A (in Massachusetts) and follow Rte. 1A south for 1.5 miles. Turn left on Armistice Blvd. and continue for 0.6 miles to the park entrance on the right. Trail access is available from the perimeter road at the opposite side of the park, as shown on the trail map.

Slater Memorial Park from I-195 eastbound: Take Exit 4 and follow Rte. 44 east for 1.5 miles. Turn left on Rte. 1A north and continue for 4.1 miles, turn right on Armistice Blvd. and drive for 0.6 miles, and turn right at the park entrance. Trail access is available from the perimeter road at the opposite side of the park, as shown on the trail map.

Kimberly Ann Rock Memorial Athletic Complex from I-195 eastbound: Take Exit 4 and follow Rte. 44 east for 1.5 miles. Turn left on Rte. 1A north and drive for 2.3 miles, then turn right on Ferris Ave. and continue for 0.5 miles to the park entrance on the left.

TOILETS:

Slater Memorial Park

ADDITIONAL INFORMATION:

Pawtucket Planning Dept., (401) 725-5200
East Providence Recreation Dept., (401) 435-7511

44 East Bay Bike Path

Providence - Bristol, RI

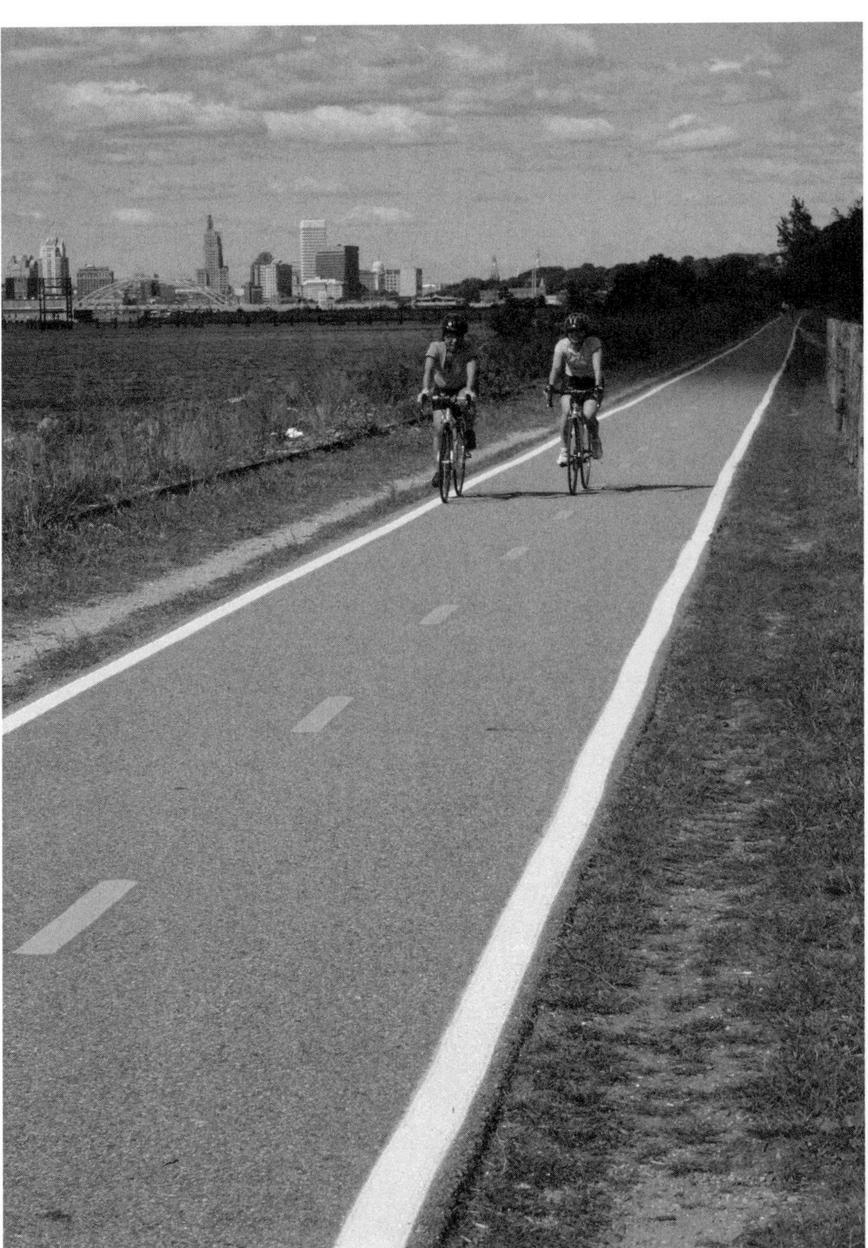

LENGTH: 14.9 miles, including short on-road bike route
SURFACE: paved
TERRAIN: flat, except for slope at Veterans Memorial Pkwy.

Rhode Island's oldest rail-trail is a sightseeing delight joining the outskirts of Providence to a string of towns, parks, and water views along the shore of Narragansett Bay.

RULES & SAFETY:

- Bicyclists should yield to pedestrians.
- Keep to the right, pass on the left, and alert others (*"On your left..."*) when approaching from behind.
- Note that walkers are asked to use the left side.
- The trail can be busy, so ride at a safe speed. Use extra caution in crowded areas and when children and pets are present since their actions can be unpredictable.
- Step off the trail when stopped to allow others to pass.
- The trail intersects many roads. Use caution before crossing streets and assume that drivers do not see you.
- Respect the private property along the trail.
- Dogs must be leashed and their wastes removed.

ORIENTATION:

The trail is exposed to wind, so note its direction when starting your ride and plan for its effects. Ideally, begin your ride heading into the wind so that the return trip will be in the easier downwind direction.

The trail ventures through populated areas and intersects a relatively large number of roads, but is well-equipped with signs, crosswalks, and traffic signal controls. Two sets of mileage markers painted on the pavement at half-mile intervals originate from both endpoints.

TRAIL DESCRIPTION:

From the **Fort Hill** trailhead in East Providence near the northern endpoint, the trail extends in two directions. Heading north (facing the trail and turning right), it runs for 1.5 miles including a short, on-road section. The ride begins with a quarter-mile descent beside **Veterans Memorial Pkwy.**, then turns left on First St. following green *Bike Route*

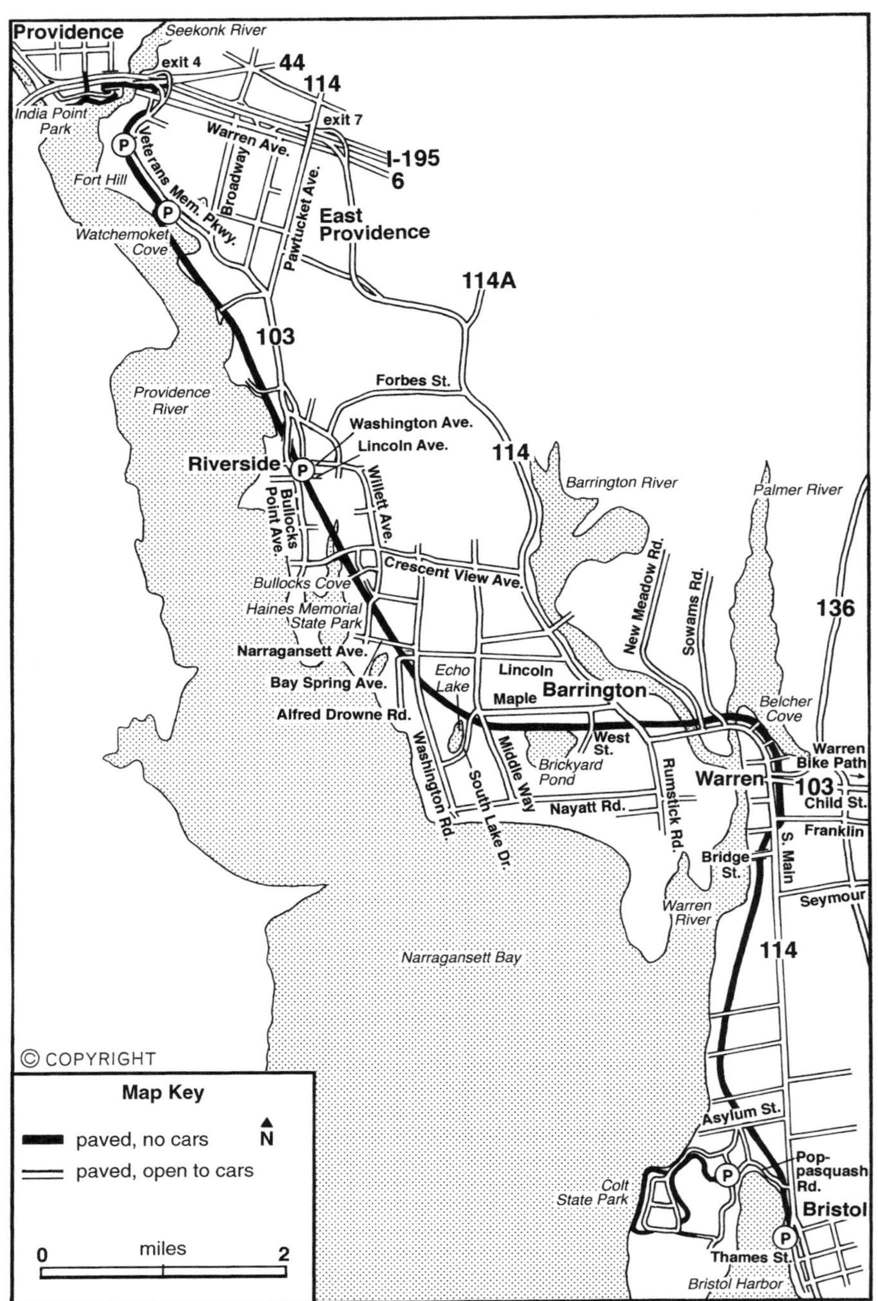

Providence
Seekonk River
exit 4
44
114
India Point Park
exit 7
Warren Ave.
I-195
6
Fort Hill
Veterans Mem. Pkwy.
Broadway
Pawtucket Ave.
East Providence
Watchemoket Cove
114A
103
Providence River
Forbes St.
Washington Ave.
Lincoln Ave.
Riverside
114
Barrington River
Palmer River
Bullocks Point Ave.
Willett Ave.
Crescent View Ave.
New Meadow Rd.
Sowams Rd.
136
Bullocks Cove
Haines Memorial State Park
Narragansett Ave.
Bay Spring Ave.
Echo Lake
Lincoln
Maple
Barrington
Belcher Cove
Alfred Drowne Rd.
West St.
Warren Bike Path
Brickyard Pond
Warren
103
Child St.
Washington Rd.
South Lake Dr.
Middle Way
Nayatt Rd.
Rumstick Rd.
Franklin
S. Main
Bridge St.
Seymour
Warren River
114
Narragansett Bay
© COPYRIGHT
Map Key
paved, no cars
paved, open to cars
N
0
miles
2
Asylum St.
Pop-pasquash Rd.
Colt State Park
Bristol
Thames St.
Bristol Harbor

signs. Ride to the end and cross **Warren Ave.** to reach the next segment of the path which climbs to the Washington Bridge and crosses the **Seekonk River** on a narrow passageway beside **I-195**.

Entering **Providence** on the other side, it descends on ramps to Gano St. and crosses to join a sidewalk curving to the right (south) beside India St. Look for a separated bike path ahead on the left entering **India Point Park** where shade trees, benches, and paved trails occupy a half-mile stretch of shoreline in front of the city. The landscaped India Point Park Bridge spans I-195 to link East St.

Heading south (left) from the Fort Hill trailhead, the trail extends for 13.4 miles. It parallels Veterans Memorial Pkwy. for the first 0.8 miles to another trailhead, then turns from the roadside and descends to a railroad bed beside the **Providence River** and a view of the city skyline. The trail emerges on a causeway separating **Watchemoket Cove** and follows the shore for the next 2 miles.

The scenery switches between shoreline and woods as the trail intersects a few private roads, then the bike path separates from the water and passes under **Bullocks Point Ave.** 3.1 miles from the Fort Hill trailhead. It intersects **Washington Ave.** (3.3 miles) at a trailhead parking lot in the village of **Riverside**, and passes a former train station before crossing **Lincoln Ave.** (3.4 miles).

Returning to tree cover, the bike path straightens through a residential area and across a causeway at the tip of **Bullocks Cove**, then intersects **Crescent View Ave.** (4.3 miles). It passes a playground at Vintner Ave. (4.6 miles) and enters Barrington at **Narragansett Ave.** (4.8 miles) and the entrance to **Haines Memorial State Park** where picnic tables, toilets, and a view of Bullocks Cove await.

Continuing southward, the trail follows a grassy, open corridor through another cluster of road intersections at **Bay Spring Ave.** (5.2 miles), **Alfred Drowne Rd.** (5.4 miles), and **Washington Rd.** (5.6 miles). It returns to woods as it slowly curves left (east) past a glimpse of **Echo Lake**, then intersects **South Lake Dr.** (6.2 miles) and **Middle Way** (6.3 miles). Another straight line brings the bike path eastward through woods at Veterans Memorial Park and along the shore of **Brickyard Pond**.

Shortly after **West St.** (7.2 miles) the trail emerges beside a shopping center in downtown Barrington and the busy intersection of **Rte. 103/114** (7.6 miles), where a cross-walk and signal await. A half-mile ahead, it enjoys water views at bridges over the **Barrington River** (8.1 miles) and **Palmer River** (8.5 miles) where it enters the town of Warren.

Turning back to the right (south), the trail has a view of **Belcher Cove** on the left before it hits another series of roads and driveways near the center of town, the busiest being **Child St.** (**Rte. 103**) (9.3 miles) and **S. Main St.** (**Rte. 114**) (9.7 miles). Signal controls are present at both.

A short distance to the east, the 0.8-mile **Warren Bike Path** offers a side trip to a view of the Kickamuit River. To find it, turn left (east) on Child St. (Rte. 103) and ride for 1 mile, turn right on Hugh Cole Rd., and look for the trail 0.4 miles ahead. Turn right on the trail to reach the river.

The East Bay Bike Path continues southward under-neath **Bridge St.** (9.9 miles) and descends past dead end residential streets to the shore of the **Warren River** where the Jacobs Point Salt Marsh spreads to the right (west). Here it hits the Bristol town line (10.7 miles) and intersects a boardwalk trail of an Audubon sanctuary. Bicycles are not permitted on the boardwalk but foot traffic is welcome.

The trail continues past shoreline homes and quiet streets for the next few miles. At the intersection of tree-lined **Asylum St.** (12.4 miles), identifiable by its separate travel lanes, turn right to reach 460-acre **Colt State Park** where several miles of paved bike paths and quiet roads explore stately grounds overlooking **Narragansett Bay**.

Continuing southward, the trail's final leg joins the shore of Mill Pond, crosses **Poppasquash Rd.** (13.1 miles), and follows **Bristol Harbor** to Independence Park on **Thames St.**, 13.4 miles from the Fort Hill trailhead.

BACKGROUND:

This route was originally the Providence, Warren & Bristol Railroad. After it was completed in 1855, the line was extended from Warren to Fall River, MA and eventually created a direct route between Providence and Newport. It had a period of strong business before the popularity of automobiles and the hardship of the Great Depression ended passenger service in the late 1930's. Freight service lasted until the 1970's, when the tracks were removed.

The East Bay Bike Path became Rhode Island's first rail-trail in 1987, and has recently been enhanced with the connection of the India Point Park Bridge in Providence. The bike path has the honor of being included in the Rails-to-Trails Conservancy's "Rail-Trail Hall of Fame" representing the nation's best rail-trails.

DRIVING DIRECTIONS:

Fort Hill trailhead, I-195 eastbound: Take Exit 4 and keep right for Riverside. Look for the first trailhead parking lot 0.4 miles ahead on the right at the top of the hill.

Fort Hill trailhead, I-195 westbound: Take Exit 6, turn left off the ramp and follow Broadway south for 1 mile. Turn right on Veterans Mem. Pkwy. and continue for 1.1 miles, then find the trailhead parking lots on the left at the top of the hill.

Riverside trailhead, I-195 eastbound: Take Exit 4 and keep right for Riverside. Follow Veterans Mem. Pkwy. south for 2.3 miles, merge onto Rte. 103 East and continue south for 1.4 miles, then turn left on Washington St.

Riverside trailhead, I-195 westbound: Take Exit 6, turn left off the ramp and follow Broadway south for 1 mile. Turn left on Veterans Mem. Pkwy. and drive for 0.8 miles, merge on Rte. 103 East and continue south for 1.4 miles, then turn left on Washington St.

Bristol trailhead: From I-195 eastbound take Exit 7 and follow Rte. 114 south for 11.6 miles. After the road comes beside Bristol Harbor, turn right on Thames St. and park at Independence Park ahead on the right.

TOILETS:

Haines Mem. State Park, Colt State Park, Independence Park

ADDITIONAL INFORMATION:

Colt State Park, (401) 253-7482

Appendix

Alliance for Biking & Walking,
P.O. Box 65150, Washington, DC 20035,
(202) 449-9692,
www.peoplepoweredmovement.org

Bike Walk Connecticut,
P.O. Box 270149, West Hartford, CT 06127,
www.bikewalkconnecticut.org

Bikes Belong Coalition
P.O. Box 2359, Boulder, CO 80306
(303) 449-4893
www.bikesbelong.org

Connecticut Dept. of Energy & Environmental Protection,
79 Elm St., Hartford, CT 06106-5127,
(860) 424-3000,
www.ct.gov/dep

East Coast Greenway Alliance,
www.greenway.org

Rails-to-Trails Conservancy,
Duke Ellington Bldg.,
2121 Ward Ct., NW, 5th Fl., Washington, DC 20037,
(202) 331-9696,
www.railstotrails.org

Rhode Island Bicycle Coalition,
ribike.org

Rhode Island Dept. of Environmental Management,
Office of Parks & Recreation,
2321 Hartford Ave., Johnston, RI 02919-1719,
(401) 222-2632,
www.dem.ri.gov or www.riparks.com